MW00845392

THE ATHLETE'S ELBOW

EDITED BY
WILLIAM N. LEVINE, MD
ASSOCIATE PROFESSOR AND VICE CHAIRMAN
DEPARTMENT OF ORTHOPAEDIC SURGERY
COLUMBIA UNIVERSITY MEDICAL CENTER
NEW YORK, NEW YORK

SERIES EDITOR
PETER C. AMADIO, MD
MAYO CLINIC
ROCHESTER, MINNESOTA

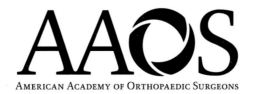

AAOS
AMERICAN ACADEMY OF ORTHOPAEDIC SURGEONS

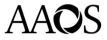

AAOS
AMERICAN ACADEMY OF
ORTHOPAEDIC SURGEONS

AMERICAN ACADEMY OF
ORTHOPAEDIC SURGEONS
BOARD OF DIRECTORS, 2008-2009

E. Anthony Rankin, MD
 President
Joseph D. Zuckerman, MD
 First Vice President
John J. Callaghan, MD
 Second Vice President
William L. Healy, MD
 Treasurer
Frederick M. Azar, MD
 Treasurer-Elect (Ex-Officio)
Thomas C. Barber, MD
Richard J. Barry, MD
James H. Beaty, MD
Kevin J. Bozic, MD, MBA
Leesa M. Galatz, MD
John T. Gill, MD
Christopher D. Harner, MD
M. Bradford Henley, MD, MBA
William J. Robb III, MD
Michael F. Schafer, MD
James P. Tasto, MD
G. Zachary Wilhoit, MS, MBA
Karen L. Hackett, FACHE, CAE *(Ex-Officio)*

STAFF

Mark W. Wieting, *Chief Education Officer*
Marilyn L. Fox, PhD, *Director, Department of
 Publications*
Laurie Braun, *Managing Editor*
Mary Steermann Bishop, *Manager, Production
 and Archives*
Courtney Astle, *Assistant Production Manager*
Susan Morritz Baim, *Production Coordinator*
Suzanne O'Reilly, *Graphics Coordinator*
Charlie Baldwin, *Page Production Assistant*
Karen Danca, *Permissions Coordinator*
Laura Khoshaba, *Publications Assistant*

The Athlete's Elbow

Published by the
American Academy of Orthopaedic Surgeons
6300 North River Road
Rosemont, IL 60018
1-800-626-6726

The material presented in *The Athlete's Elbow* has been made available by the American Academy of Orthopaedic Surgeons for educational purposes only. This material is not intended to present the only, or necessarily best, methods or procedures for the medical situations discussed, but rather is intended to represent an approach, view, statement, or opinion of the author(s) or producer(s), which may be helpful to others who face similar situations.

Some drugs or medical devices demonstrated in Academy courses or described in Academy print or electronic publications have not been cleared by the Food and Drug Administration (FDA) or have been cleared for specific uses only. The FDA has stated that it is the responsibility of the physician to determine the FDA clearance status of each drug or device he or she wishes to use in clinical practice.

Furthermore, any statements about commercial products are solely the opinion(s) of the author(s) and do not represent an Academy endorsement or evaluation of these products. These statements may not be used in advertising or for any commercial purpose.

All rights reserved. No part of this publication may be reproduced, stored in a retrieval system, or transmitted, in any form, or by any means, electronic, mechanical, photocopying, recording, or otherwise, without prior written permission from the publisher.

First Edition
Copyright © 2008 by the
American Academy of Orthopaedic Surgeons

ISBN 10: 0-89203-455-6
ISBN 13: 978-0-89203-455-0

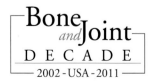

Bone *and* Joint
D E C A D E
2002 - USA - 2011

CONTRIBUTORS

Christopher S. Ahmad, MD
Assistant Professor
Center for Shoulder, Elbow, and Sports
  Medicine
Department of Orthopaedic Surgery
Columbia University
New York, NY

Theodore A. Blaine, MD
Associate Professor
Brown Alpert Medical School
University Orthopedics, Inc.
Rhode Island Hospital and
  The Miriam Hospital
Providence, RI

John E. Conway, MD
Private Practice
Fort Worth, TX

Neal ElAttrache, MD[a]
Director, Sports Medicine Fellowship
Kerlan-Jobe Orthopaedic Clinic
Associate Clinical Professor, Department of
  Orthopaedics
Keck School of Medicine, University of
  Southern California
Los Angeles, CA

Guillem Gonzalez-Lomas, MD
Resident
Department of Orthopaedic Surgery
Columbia University
New York, NY

Matthew A. Kippe, MD
Orthopaedic Surgery Consultant
Hawthorn Medical Associates
St. Luke's Hospital
North Dartmouth, MA

William N. Levine, MD
Associate Professor and Vice Chairman
Department of Orthopaedic Surgery
Columbia University Medical Center
New York, NY

Derek Moore, MD
Fellow
Orthopaedic Spine Surgery
Hospital for Special Surgery
New York, NY

Bernard F. Morrey, MD
Professor of Orthopedic Surgery
Department of Orthopedics
Mayo Clinic
Rochester, MN

Duong Nguyen, MD, FRCSC
Orthopedic Surgery Consultant
Sports Medicine, Shoulder, and Elbow Center
OrthoCarolina
Charlotte, NC

Shawn W. O'Driscoll, PhD, MD
Professor of Orthopedic Surgery
Department of Orthopedics
Mayo Clinic
Rochester, MN

CONTRIBUTORS (CONT.)

Jonathan D. Packer, MD
Department of Orthopaedic Surgery
Columbia University
New York, NY

Daniel E. Prince, MD, MPH
New York Presbyterian – Columbia University
New York, NY

Robert Z. Tashjian, MD
Assistant Professor
Department of Orthopaedics
University of Utah School of Medicine
Salt Lake City, UT

Ken Yamaguchi, MD[b]
Sam and Marilyn Fox Distinguished Professor
Washington University Orthopedics
Washington University School of Medicine
St. Louis, MO

a. Neal ElAttrache, MD or the department with which he is affiliated has received research or institutional support and royalties from Arthrex.
b. Ken Yamaguchi, MD or the department with which he is affiliated has received research or institutional support and royalties from Tornier, Zimmer, and Arthrex.

CONTENTS

PREFACE

Advances in the understanding and management of elbow problems have increased dramatically over the last decade. *The Athlete's Elbow* provides a state-of-the art review of common problems encountered in the management of elbow pathology in athletes and other patients. Recognized leaders in the field have brought their insights and experience to each of the chapters. The latest advances in physical examination tests, preoperative diagnostic tests, and arthroscopic and open techniques are highlighted throughout the monograph.

It is my hope that this monograph will serve as a reference for orthopaedic surgeons, residents, fellows, sports medicine experts, primary care physicians, and allied health professionals to help guide the care and management of elbow disorders in pediatric and adult patients.

I would like to thank the contributing authors who have donated their valuable time to this project because of their shared passion for education, teaching, and pushing the envelope with basic science and clinical research. I would also like to thank Marilyn Fox, PhD, Director of the Department of Publications; and Laurie Braun, Managing Editor, who have helped see this project through to completion. Finally, and perhaps most importantly, I would like to thank my wife, Jill, and daughters, Sonya Belle and Clare Simone, for allowing me to pursue my academic interests (usually late at night and on weekends!) and for their unwavering love and support.

William N. Levine, MD
Editor

CHAPTER 1

PEDIATRIC AND ADOLESCENT SPORTS ELBOW INJURIES

CHRISTOPHER S. AHMAD, MD
GUILLEM GONZALEZ-LOMAS, MD

BACKGROUND/EPIDEMIOLOGY

In the last few decades, the young athlete has been thrust into an athletic environment that demands an increasing amount of training and performance at a young age. In the United States, 35 million children and young adults between the ages of 6 and 20 years participate in sports. Each year, more than 3.5 million sports-related injuries in children younger than age 15 years are treated in hospitals, offices, clinics, and emergency departments. This increased participation in sports has led to a concomitant increase in upper extremity and elbow injuries. For example, baseball players 9 to 12 years of age have a 20% to 40% annual incidence of elbow pain.[1,2]

The physis is generally considered to be the weak link in the elbow of the skeletally immature athlete, but muscular, tendinous, and other bony injuries also occur. The specific demands of a sport may induce certain injury patterns to predominate. For example, in sports in which the elbow bears constant, repetitive strain, such as baseball and gymnastics, overuse syndromes preferentially arise. By contrast, in high-contact sports like football or hockey, impact injuries leading to fractures occur more frequently. The orthopaedic surgeon must keep in mind the anatomy, sport-specific biomechanics, and unique pathology of the immature elbow when treating the young athlete.

ANATOMY

The elbow is a diarthrodial joint in which the distal humerus articulates with the proximal ulna and the radial head. Its unique bony configuration allows for −15° to 0° of extension and 150° of flexion. Rotation of the radial head over the stationary ulna gives an arc of nearly 180° of forearm rotation.[3] In young children, the structures that comprise the elbow are primarily cartilaginous. Knowledge of the pattern of the radiographic appearance and closure of elbow ossification centers helps differentiate normal anatomy from fractures or avulsions.

The mnemonic CRITOE (capitellum, age 2; radial head, age 4; internal [medial] epicondyle, age 6; trochlea, age 7; olecranon, age 9; and external [lateral] epicondyle, age 10) can facilitate recall of the order of secondary ossification center appearance. In boys, the centers appear roughly 6 to 12 months later than in girls. All the ossification centers fuse at puberty (in girls, at 14 to 15 years of age; in boys, at 15 to 17 years).

Because 80% of longitudinal growth of the arm occurs at the proximal humerus, growth at the elbow is generally only appositional, through the apophyses. In addition, the physes of the elbow are inherently weaker than the bones and ligaments surrounding them. Excessive forces on the ligaments and tendons inserting into the apophyses often avulse the apophyses before the tendon or ligament is torn.

In full extension, the elbow hangs at a normal valgus angle of 11° to 16°. Elbow stability is governed by bony geometry, ligamentous restraints, and muscular dynamic restraints. The bone and articular congruency of the humerus, ulna, and radial head account for the greater part of elbow stability, particularly at less than 20° of extension or more than 120° of elbow flexion.[4] In the arc of 20° to 120° of elbow flexion, however—the arc of the throwing motion—ligamentous restraints provide primary stability, although the bony elbow structures still provide critical stability.[5] Ligamentous restraints include the anterior joint capsule, the ulnar collateral ligament (UCL) complex, and the lateral collateral ligament (LCL) complex. For example, controversy still exists as to how much valgus strain the olecranon unloads off the UCL.[6-8] Dynamic stabilizers include the flexor carpi ulnaris and the flexor digitorum superficialis.[9]

The UCL complex consists of three ligaments: the anterior oblique bundle, the posterior oblique bundle, and a variable transverse oblique bundle.[8] Of these, the anterior bundle, which is composed of an anterior and posterior band, provides the greatest stabilizing resistance to valgus stress from 30° to 120° of flexion.[5] As such, it serves a crucial stabilizing role in the overhead throwing athlete. It must withstand near-failure tensile stresses during the acceleration phase of the throwing motion.[8]

The LCL complex contains three major ligamentous structures: the radial collateral ligament, the lateral UCL, and the accessory collateral ligament. The lateral UCL protects against rotatory subluxation of the ulnohumeral joint. If the lateral UCL is injured, posterolateral rotatory instability ensues. The radial collateral ligament has been purported to act as an important secondary restraint of the lateral elbow along with the extensor muscles, including the extensor digitorum communis, the brachioradialis, and the extensor carpi radialis longus and brevis.

The skeletally immature elbow differs from its adult counterpart in that it possesses a greater degree of cartilaginous elasticity. This affects injuries to the elbow in two ways. First, its young, thick, cartilage-laden joint surfaces lack the rigid congruency of an adult elbow. The coronoid and olecranon do not "lock in" as rigidly during flexion and extension. This play, coupled with an increased intrinsic capsular laxity, allows children to hyperextend their elbows between 10° and 15°. Consequently, the pediatric elbow dislocates more often without an associated fracture. If the elbow subsequently spontaneously reduces, the only signs of dislocation may be pain and swelling.

Second, the ability of the elbow to hyperextend also places more compressive load laterally, on the radiocapitellar joint, and stretches out the medial capsule and

UCL. Overhead throwing athletes further exaggerate these stresses during the throwing motion. Repetitive stress on this system can lead to osteochondritis/osteochondrosis of lateral structures such as the radial head or capitellum and medial-sided pathology such as medial apophysitis from the excessive valgus stress.[10]

BIOMECHANICS OF THROWING

The six phases of throwing, depicted in **Figure 1**, include windup, early cocking, late cocking, acceleration, deceleration, and follow-through. The preeminent characteristics of the throwing motion are a large valgus load (generated by a varus torque) and rapid extension. During the late cocking phase, elbow varus torques as high as 64 N·m have been registered in adults. More typically, a 73-mph fastball will generate 44 N·m of varus torque, of which about half will be absorbed by the UCL.[11] In the acceleration phase, the elbow reaches an angular velocity of 3,000°/s as it extends from around 110° to 20°.[11] The combination of the valgus load and rapid extension generates three major stresses: a tensile stress along medial restraints (UCL, flexor pronator mass, medial epicondyle apophysis, and ulnar nerve), a shear stress in the posterior compartment (posteromedial tip of olecranon and trochlea/olecranon fossa), and a compression stress laterally in the radiocapitellar joint of up to 500 N. Each stress can cause pathology, either acutely or from overuse. The medial tensile stress in the skeletally immature athlete can lead to medial apophysitis. Other injuries, including UCL sprain, ulnar neuritis, medial epicondylitis, and pronator mass tendinitis, occur more frequently in older adolescents with closed physes. In the posterior compartment, the olecranon tip and olecranon fossa may develop osteophytes. Osteophytes in the olecranon tip can cause impingement on the posteromedial trochlea, leading to a "kissing" lesion of chondromalacia. This constellation of medial, posterior, and lateral compartment elbow injuries has been called valgus extension overload syndrome.[12] **Figure 2** illustrates the injuries that comprise valgus extension overload syndrome.

Children throw similarly to adults, with very comparable kinematics.[13-15] Some differences do exist, however. One study comparing Little League, adolescent, and college/professional pitchers found that the younger Little League players generated slower trunk, hip rotation, and

FIGURE 1

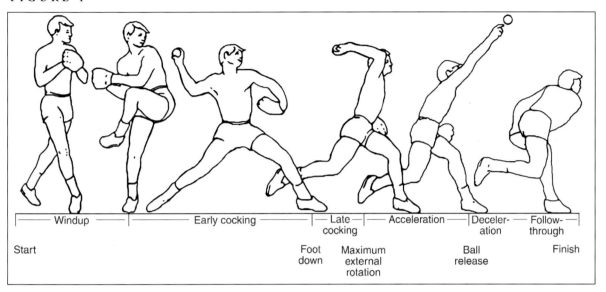

Windup — Early cocking — Late cocking — Acceleration — Decel-eration — Follow-through

Start   Foot down   Maximum external rotation   Ball release   Finish

Phases of overhead throwing. (Reproduced with permission from Fleisig GS, Barrentine SW, Escamilla RF, Andrews JR: Biomechanics of overhand throwing with implications for injuries. *Sports Med* 1996;21:421-437.)

shoulder external rotation velocities; had increased horizontal adduction in the cocking phase and less arm abduction during acceleration; and generally did not synchronize the arm motion with the body. Some players compensated for their different kinematics by developing a throwing motion more akin to throwing a dart. Interestingly, although this motion represents poor form, it generates lower forces and torque than that of better players who throw faster,[14] and the result is relatively protective.[13]

Different pitches can also produce more or less torque on the elbow. Escamilla and associates[16] showed that the fastball and slider produced the highest forces on the shoulder and elbow. The curveball generated the highest elbow valgus stress. Recently, Fleisig and associates[17] examined collegiate baseball pitchers and showed that the change-up produced less torque on the elbow and was thus safer than either the curveball or the fastball. These results are in adults, however, and have not been studied in children or adolescents. Nevertheless, better Little League players tend to be the ones who pitch fastballs and curveballs. In addition, they generally pitch more often, on more teams, and with better form. These factors conspire to further overload the elbow and make it more vulnerable to injury. At this time, the best way to mitigate injury is to limit the volume of pitching.[18]

IMAGING

AP and lateral radiographs should be obtained routinely, especially to rule out physeal injuries or avulsion fractures, even when overwhelming evidence of ligamentous injury exists. Several radiographic relationships characterize proper alignment of the elbow. First, the midaxial line of the radius should bisect the capitellum on all views. Second, the anterior humeral line should extend through the middle third of the capitellum. An anterior fat pad sign is often physiologic, but a posterior fat pad sign almost always connotes a fracture. Skaggs and Mirzayan[19] showed that 76% of patients who had no radiographic signs of fracture but did have a posterior fat pad sign were found to have a fracture upon follow-up 3 weeks later. Therefore, these patients should be treated as if they have a nondisplaced fracture about the elbow. Contralateral comparison views should always be obtained.

If there is no overt fracture but a ligamentous injury is suspected, a stress view should be obtained. This may show a physeal fracture (which will often occur before any ligament damage) or opening up of the joint. MRI scans or sonograms may be obtained to assess ligament injuries that will be manifested by discontinuation of the UCL or aberrations in the anatomy. Finally, dynamic sonography can be used to visualize valgus

FIGURE 2

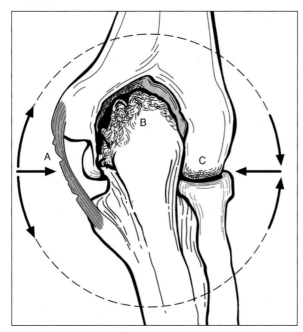

Schematic of posteromedial impingement as a part of valgus extension overload syndrome. A shows the area of medial tension stress on the UCL, B indicates posteromedial impingement with olecranon osteophytes, and C is lateral compression injury to the radiocapitellar joint. The arrows indicate tension and compression forces. (Reproduced with permission from ElAttrache NS, Ahmad CS: Valgus extension overload and olecranon stress fractures. *Sports Med Arthrosc Rev* 2003;11:25-29.)

joint instability in UCL injuries while the elbow is being stressed.[20]

INJURIES

In general, injury should be suspected with pain at rest, pain at night, increasing pain despite rest, and pain refractory to treatment with ice and other modalities.

Lateral Elbow Pain

Panner Disease
Panner disease, defined as osteochondrosis of the capitellum, was first described in 1927 by Panner,[21] who identified its similarities to Legg-Calvé-Perthes disease. Like all other osteochondroses, Panner disease is described as noninflammatory, disordered endochondral ossification. Although its specific etiology and relationship to osteochondritis dissecans (OCD) remain debatable, most authors agree that it results from abnormal compressive forces placed over the radiocapitellar joint during a period of vulnerability.[22-24] Its etiology likely includes an avascular component, the result of a predominantly end-artery supply to the capitellum in combination with repetitive microtrauma.[25] In general, Panner disease affects children younger than age 10 years.[26] Young boys tend to be predisposed to this condition for two reasons: (1) The delayed appearance and maturation of secondary growth centers in boys, and (2) their susceptibility to trauma during early childhood activities.[23] Distinctively, Panner disease does not share the strict association with repetitive throwing that OCD does, is usually self-limiting, and classically resolves without any long-term sequelae.

Patients with Panner disease initially present with pain and stiffness in the elbow that is relieved by rest. Physical examination reveals poorly localized tenderness over the lateral elbow. Radiographs initially show fissuring and irregularity of the capitellum as seen in **Figure 3**, but subsequent films demonstrate reossification with a corresponding resolution of symptoms. Treatment involves rest from the offending activity and alleviating modalities such as ice and nonsteroidal anti-inflammatory drugs as needed. The elbow may sometimes need to be immobilized for 3 to 4 weeks. Although symptoms can persist for months, the condition has an excellent long-term prognosis.

Osteochondritis Dissecans
OCD is much more common in the immature athlete than in the adult. In the elbow, OCD preferentially involves the capitellum. It is believed to be a noninflammatory degeneration of the subchondral bone. There may be a relationship between Panner disease and OCD. Some authors have even proposed that the two conditions are two different stages of the same disorder.[27] Nevertheless, the two conditions can be differentiated by age of onset, etiology, and natural history. Panner affects younger children, whereas OCD is more common in older athletes, between the ages of 11 and 15 years.[15] Unlike Panner, OCD is thought to be directly linked to repetitive trauma and is not self-limiting. If left unaddressed, it results in profound destruction of the capitellum.[15]

OCD arises from repetitive, excessive compressive forces generated by large valgus stresses on the elbow when a ball is thrown or a racket swung, and from constant axial compressive loads on the elbow in the gymnast.[15,28,29] Specific risk factors predispose to the condition.

FIGURE 3

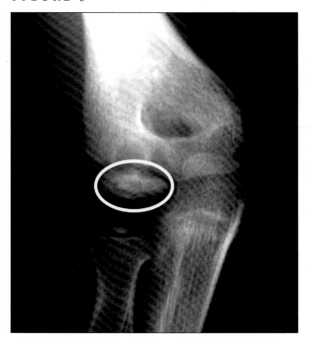

AP radiograph showing Panner disease. The circle highlights the area of fissuring in the capitellum.

FIGURE 4

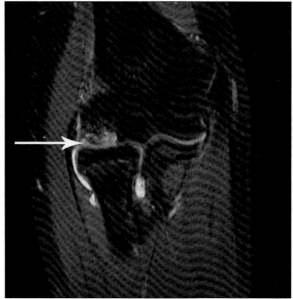

Coronal MRI of the elbow of a 14-year-old female gymnast with OCD of the capitellum (arrow).

In baseball players, throwing sliders and breaking pitches, throwing more than 600 pitches per season, and advanced age of the athlete increase the risk of developing OCD.[29] Overtraining and excessive elbow compressive stress (eg, handstands) have also been linked to OCD in the female gymnast.[30,31] Other risk factors include genetic predisposition and the tenuous end-artery vascular supply to the capitellum. The capitellum is supplied by two end arteries coursing from posterior to anterior (the radial recurrent and interosseous recurrent arteries.) Blood flow to the capitellum may be disrupted during repetitive microtrauma, resulting in an avascular state that may initiate OCD. A single traumatic event may also predispose to the development of OCD as a sequela of posttraumatic subchondral bone bruises.[32]

Patients with OCD initially present with pain and stiffness in the elbow that is relieved by rest. If left unaddressed, the symptoms progress to "locking" or "catching" due to intra-articular loose bodies. Physical examination is remarkable for lateral elbow tenderness, usually poorly localized over the radiocapitellar joint. Range of motion is usually limited, with loss of extension more common than loss of flexion. A positive active radiocapitellar compression test suggests radiocapitellar joint pathology. In this test, pronating and supinating the forearm with the arm in extension elicits pain.

Radiographs may be negative early in the disease process, but flattening and sclerosis of the capitellum, classically on the anterolateral aspect of the capitellum, are seen later. Irregular areas of lucency as well as intra-articular loose bodies also appear and are best seen on AP radiographs with 45° elbow flexion. In suspected OCD, MRI should always be obtained (**Figure 4**). It will detect bone edema early in the disease process.[33] MR arthrography can further delineate the extent of the injury. The contrast can show separation of a detached piece from subchondral bone. Occasionally, a pseudolesion on the posteroinferior aspect of the capitellum can be mistaken for OCD, but true OCD occurs on the anterolateral aspect.

An MRI classification and an arthroscopic classification that correlate with each other have been developed, and they can be used to guide treatment.[34] **Table 1** summarizes both classifications. In type IA, radiographs are negative; T1-weighted MRI is abnormal, but T2-weighted images are normal. Arthroscopically, the articular cartilage is intact with no loss of subchondral stability. This

---

TABLE 1

MRI and Arthroscopic Classifications of OCD

MRI-Based Classification		Arthroscopic-Based Classification	
Type	MRI Findings	Type	Arthroscopic Findings
IA	Normal radiograph T1: abnormal signal in superficial capitellum Normal T2	Intact/stable	Intact articular cartilage/ subchondral stability intact
IB	Abnormal radiograph T1 and T2: abnormal signal	Intact/unstable	Intact articular cartilage/ unstable subchondral bone with impending collapse
II	MRI with contrast shows margin around lesion	Open/unstable	Cartilage fracture/subchondral bone collapse or displacement
III	Chronic lesions with loose bodies	Detached	Loose bodies
IV	Associated radial head OCD		

Adapted with permission from Voloshin I, Schena A: Elbow Injuries, in Schepsis AA, Busconi BD (eds): *Sports Medicine*. Philadelphia, PA, Lippincott Williams and Wilkins, 2006.

---

stage, defined as early OCD, can be treated conservatively. All activity involving the affected arm should be stopped. The elbow should be rested in a hinged elbow brace for 3 to 6 weeks, followed by nonsteroidal anti-inflammatory drugs (NSAIDs) and progressive physical therapy as symptoms abate. Return to sport usually can be expected at 3 to 6 months. Follow-up radiographs should also be obtained at 3 to 6 months. Notably, radiographic changes often lag behind the clinical symptoms by several months or years, so return to sports should be governed by clinical response. If symptoms return, additional rest is mandated. With persistently refractory symptoms, pitchers may have to change positions and gymnasts may have to change sports.

In type IB lesions, abnormal signal is seen on both T1- and T2-weighted MRI. Arthroscopically, the cartilage is intact, but the subchondral bone is unstable and ready to collapse. Treatment should initially parallel that for a type IA lesion. If this fails, the size and orientation of the lesion governs the treatment. Lesions affecting <55% of the capitellum and with <60° angle on the lateral radiograph have been treated with subchondral drilling with some success.[35] Larger lesions should be fixed with metallic or bioabsorbable implants. Of note, lesions affecting ≥70%

of the capitellum and with >90° angle on the lateral radiograph have a poor outcome. If the lesion is chronic, as documented by an old MRI scan or by arthroscopic assessment, it should be débrided and drilled. Mosaicplasty (osteochondral autologous transplantation) has been recently applied in the context of elbow OCD lesions. In this procedure, small, cylindrical osteochondral grafts are obtained from the lateral periphery of the femoral condyles and transplanted to prepared osteochondral defects. Iwasaki and associates[36] obtained good or excellent results with this method in seven out of eight teenaged baseball players with OCD. If autograft is unavailable, allograft or synthetic scaffolding can be used. Closed-wedge osteotomy of the lateral distal humerus has also been used for early OCD lesions to unload the lateral compartment of the elbow. Kiyoshige and associates[37] performed a closed-wedge osteotomy developed by Yoshizu[38] 2 cm proximal to the lateral epicondyle with a 10° intervening angle in seven male baseball pitchers 7 to 12 years of age and obtained good results and a return to baseball in six of the seven patients.

In type II lesions, MRI shows a margin around the lesion, denoting its instability. Arthroscopically, the cartilage is fractured and the subchondral bone is unstable

FIGURE 5

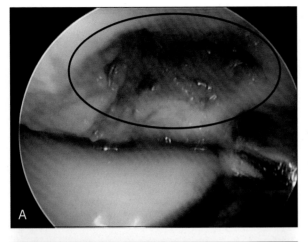

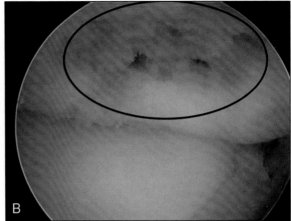

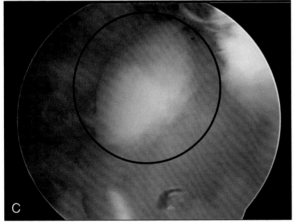

Arthroscopic views of OCD type III (loose body) lesion. **A,** Capitellar defect (inside circle) before drilling. **B,** Lesion after drilling. **C,** Loose body.

and partially displaced. When a type II lesion is identified, nonsurgical treatment should be bypassed. It warrants immediate surgical treatment with the above methods.

Type III lesions are severe, chronic lesions with loose bodies (**Figure 5**). If the loose body is shown to be acutely displaced in a patient with previously documented OCD, one can attempt to fix it to its donor site. Otherwise, loose bodies should be removed and the donor bed débrided. These patients will often be unable to return to sports. Another type III lesion is shown in **Figure 6**. In this case, the lesion was treated with a mosaicplasty. The site of the defect was prepared (**Figure 6**, *B*), then filled with a donor allograft plug (**Figure 6**, *C*).

Type IV lesions, characterized by associated radial head OCD in addition to capitellar pathology, do not generally occur in athletes. If the radial lesion is <30% of the radial head, then treatment of the capitellar OCD should proceed. For larger radial lesions, débridement, drilling, and microfracture of the capitellum are appropriate.[26]

Postoperatively, all patients should be protected for 2 to 3 weeks with a long arm cast or hinged brace. Active motion should not be started until bony union is seen on radiographs. Return to sport is usually 6 months after surgery.

Prognosis for OCD of the capitellum is good when diagnosed early, at the type IA stage. Unfortunately, most cases are diagnosed at type IB or II stages. These patients have a less favorable long-term outcome. Osteoarthritis will develop in 50% of radiocapitellar OCD patients.[39] For athletes with open physes, prevention is the best treatment. Pitch counts should be monitored and kept under 600/week. Players should never pitch or play when in pain and should never be medicated to play.

FIGURE 6

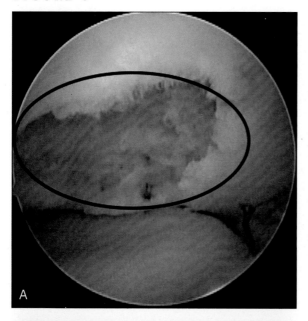

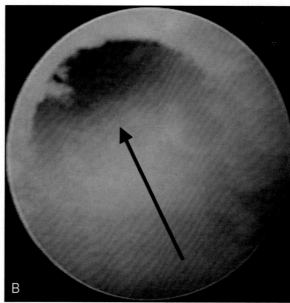

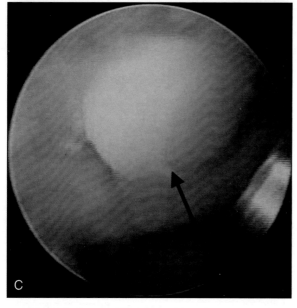

Arthroscopic views of type III capitellar OCD treated with mosaicplasty. **A**, OCD lesion (circled). **B**, Prepared tunnel; arrow points into tunnel. **C**, Arrow points to donor plug.

Medial Elbow Pain

Medial Epicondylar Apophysitis (Little League Elbow)

The term Little League elbow has recently been applied to a plethora of medial elbow injuries including medial epicondylar avulsion, medial epicondylar apophysitis, accelerated apophyseal growth with delayed closure of epicondylar growth plate, and even OCD.[40] Classically, the term refers to an apophysitis of the medial epicondylar growth plate found in skeletally immature athletes. Although the injury is more common among young baseball players, it also occurs in football quarterbacks and tennis players. In skeletally mature high school throwers, the UCL bears the brunt of the valgus stress and is preferentially injured. By contrast, in skeletally immature athletes, injury to the medial apophysis is more common.[41] The diagnosis is primarily clinical. Patients report a gradually increasing onset of medial elbow pain and stiffness, particularly when throwing. Eventually, they experience a decrease in throwing velocity and effectiveness.

The differential diagnosis for medial elbow pain includes avulsion fractures, medial epicondylitis, UCL sprain or tear, ulnar neuritis, and C8/T1 radiculopathy. Medial tenderness and swelling over the epicondyle and occasionally a flexion contracture on physical examination suggests medial epicondylar apophysitis. Early in the disease process, plain radiographs are negative in up to 85% of patients.[42] Occasionally they reveal irregular ossification of the medial epicondylar apophysis. Left untreated, the apophysis may widen, separate, and even fragment. Of note, lateral compressive injuries such as Panner disease or OCD can coexist with any medial distraction overuse injury. The most critical component of the initial management is resting the affected arm from pitching for a minimum of 4 to 6 weeks. Other conditioning activities, particularly core strengthening, should be encouraged.[43] Adjunctive ice and NSAID therapy can relieve symptoms and hasten recovery. In patients with elbow contractures, an elbow extension brace can prove beneficial. Refractory symptoms usually result from inadequate rest. In this situation, a brace or splint can be used to more definitively rest the elbow. After the initial 4 to 6 weeks of pitching abstinence, a slowly progressive throwing program is instituted over the next 6 to 8 weeks. If clinical symptoms reemerge, the athlete should stop throwing activities immediately and rest for 2 to 3 days, and then continue the therapy program. The average time to return to competitive pitching is 12 weeks. Prevention remains the optimal strategy for mitigating the incidence of the disorder. Identifying problematic throwing mechanics and correcting them can improve the prognosis. The number or type of pitches thrown can be tailored to decrease the incidence of recurrence. Lyman and associates[29] found that pitches per game and per season correlated with elbow pain in 9- to 14-year-old athletes, but poor pitching mechanics did not.

Nonsurgical management routinely succeeds for chronic medial apophysitis. If it fails, resection of the symptomatic medial epicondyle has been advocated.

However, long-term outcomes (>30 years) of epicondyle resection appear to be poor.[44] If the medial epicondyle physis widens more than 3 to 5 mm, open reduction and internal fixation with either smooth Kirschner wires (K-wires) or a T-nail appears to yield good results.[44]

Medial Epicondyle Fractures

Acute avulsions of the medial epicondyle can occur in skeletally immature athletes as a result of overwhelming valgus loads during throwing or as a result of trauma. Fractures through the medial epicondyle physis occur during adolescence. Half of the cases occur with an associated elbow dislocation; 15% of the time, the fragment gets incarcerated in the joint.[45] Displacement of the fracture guides treatment. Minimally displaced fractures can be treated by immobilization at 90° for 2 to 3 weeks followed by range-of-motion exercises. Fractures with >5 mm displacement also appear to do well with long arm cast immobilization, even if the epicondylar fragment goes on to nonunion, although immobilization carries a risk of loss of elbow joint extension.[46,47] These displaced fractures do, however, require valgus stability testing. If the fracture is unstable to valgus stress testing demonstrated by a valgus stress radiograph under anesthesia, open reduction is recommended. K-wires, sutures, and screws have all been used for fixation. Case and Hennrikus[47] used 4.5-mm cannulated screws with washers in eight adolescent athletes and obtained excellent results and return to sports in all patients. **Figure 7** shows a medial apophyseal fracture with the fractured piece visible in the ulnohumeral joint. In this case, the joint was grossly unstable. Open reduction and internal fixation with two cancellous screws restored the medial piece to its original location (**Figure 7**, *C* and *D*).

Ulnar Collateral Ligament Injuries

UCL injuries are uncommon in skeletally immature athletes. The UCL is vulnerable to repeated valgus stresses in overhead throwing athletes and stick- or racket-wielding athletes in sports like tennis and hockey. Chronic, attritional tears of the UCL almost never occur in children. If a tear is present, it is almost exclusively acute.

Patients report pain and an inability to continue performing at their prior level. Pitchers, for example, often describe losing "pop" or "zip" on the ball. The patient may remember a single episode of giving way of the medial elbow. When asked, athletes will describe the pain

FIGURE 7

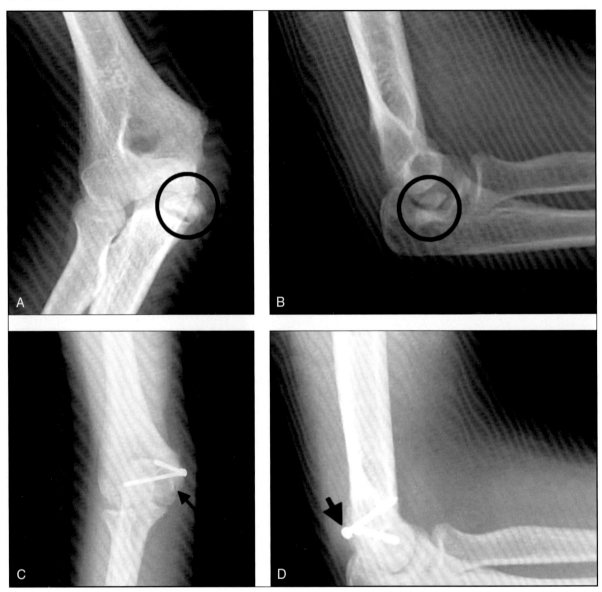

Medial epicondylar fracture. AP **(A)** and lateral **(B)** views show the fractured piece in the ulnohumeral joint, circled. AP **(C)** and lateral **(D)** views after open reduction and internal fixation with cancellous screws. Arrows point to reduction.

as worst during the acceleration phase of throwing with pain at ball release.

Physical examination may reveal a flexion contracture. In addition, patients will have point tenderness to palpation medially, usually 2 cm distal to the medial epicondyle, and pain and instability with valgus stress testing. Three methods of testing valgus stability are the valgus stress test, the milking maneuver, and the moving valgus stress test.[8] The classic valgus stress technique involves stabilizing the humerus and applying a valgus force at 30° of elbow flexion. The flexion removes the stabilizing contribution of the ulnohumeral articulation. During the milking maneuver, the athlete recreates a valgus stress by bending the affected elbow past 90° in supination, then taking the thumb with the contralateral hand and pulling down, producing a valgus-downward force. The examiner palpates the UCL to assess for tenderness and medial joint space widening. In the modified milking maneuver, the athlete places the contralateral hand under the humerus. This eliminates external rotation as a confounding motion. The examiner then pulls the thumb down with the elbow at 70° of flexion (the position of greatest valgus laxity when the UCL is sectioned in a cadaveric model).[8] The examiner's other hand palpates the medial structures for tenderness and subtle joint-space widening (≥2 mm compared to the contralateral elbow). The moving valgus stress test has recently been added to the armamentarium of UCL injury diagnostics. In this test, the patient's shoulder is placed in an abducted and externally rotated position. The elbow is then flexed and extended while a valgus force is imparted to the elbow. Athletes with UCL insufficiency will feel pain at a specific and reproducible point within the arc of 8° to 120°, reproducing the pain of throwing.[48]

Absence of pain with resisted wrist flexion will help differentiate UCL injury from flexor pronator muscle injury (medial epicondylitis/apophysitis). However, both may occur at the same time. In an acute UCL tear, the athlete may also have avulsed the flexor-pronator group. This will manifest itself as weak wrist flexion. Athletes may also present with concurrent ulnar neuritis. In those cases, symptoms that are early in the disease course (such as hand clumsiness or heaviness worsened by overhead activity, as well as tingling in the small and ring fingers) will develop. Pain may radiate from the medial elbow up the ulnar side of the forearm. Chronic insufficiency of the UCL may lead to injuries to other secondary stabilizing structures. These include flexor tendinitis, ulnar neuritis, medial apophysitis, medial epicondylitis, lateral column (radiocapitellar) compression, and loose bodies.

Plain radiographs will rarely show signs of UCL injuries, as they do in adult athletes. Stress radiographs with anesthesia can be diagnostic, but medial opening tends to be very subtle, often 2 to 3 mm. MRI is helpful in diagnosing UCL injury and can reveal injury to other secondary structures. MR arthrography has been reported to be 97% sensitive in detecting UCL injury. Diagnostic arthroscopy can visualize the medial compartment, but most of the UCL is not visualized.

Initial treatment involves rest, NSAIDs, and physical therapy for 6 weeks, with gradual progression of activ-

ity. Barnes and Tullos[49] found that half their athletes were able to return to competition with nonsurgical management. In general, 6 months are usually required before return to competition. Stability should be reassessed about 6 weeks after injury. For acute, complete UCL tears in an athlete who seeks to return to a sport that will place valgus stress on the elbow, surgical intervention is an option. Surgical treatment can include internal fixation of an avulsed fragment in the very rare cases in which it is present. Otherwise, UCL reconstruction via autograft should proceed following the same guidelines as in adults.[50] Autograft options include using the palmaris longus, fourth toe extensor, hamstring tendon, or strip of Achilles. Argo and associates[51] recently reported on surgical treatment of UCL insufficiency in 19 young women (age range, 15 to 37.5 years). They found that all had good or excellent results at mean 3-year follow-up with either plication, primary repair to bone using anchors, or palmaris graft.[51] Petty and associates[52] found that the success rate of UCL reconstruction in adolescent baseball players was almost identical to that in their adult counterparts, with 74% of players returning to baseball at the same or a higher level.[52]

Postoperatively, the elbow is immobilized for 1 week in 30° of flexion to allow the skin and soft tissues to heal, after which active wrist, elbow, and shoulder range of motion are initiated. At 4 to 6 weeks, full range-of-motion strengthening exercises begin. At 8 weeks, plyometrics are introduced. Patients with open physes are at risk for postoperative premature closure of the medial epicondylar apophysis; however, because the apophysis does not contribute to longitudinal growth, this is usually clinically irrelevant.

Posterior Elbow Pain

Olecranon Apophyseal Injury

The triceps contracts forcefully on the olecranon during the acceleration phase of throwing. In children with open physes, the strong triceps contractions pull perpendicular to the olecranon apophysis, causing a shear distracting force. Repeated bouts of powerful triceps contraction can ultimately result in olecranon apophysitis. In adolescents with closed physes, stress fractures of the olecranon apophysis occur instead.

Gore and associates[53] theorized that the disorder in question was a traction apophysitis. Other authors have compared olecranon apophysitis to Osgood-Schlatter

FIGURE 8

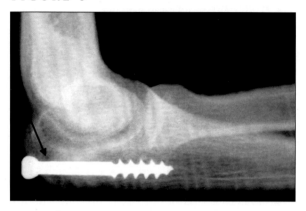

Lateral radiograph showing olecranon stress fracture after open reduction and internal fixation with intramedullary screw. Arrow points to stress fracture reduced with screw.

disease. There are reports of separated secondary olecranon ossification centers persisting into adulthood. Patients present with weakness, chronic pain, decreased range of motion, and swelling over the posterior elbow. Symptoms are worse during the acceleration and follow-through phases of throwing. Physical examination findings include tenderness over the olecranon and pain with resisted extension. In addition, valgus instability may lead to posterior compartment impingement. Radiographs classically show widening or fragmentation of the olecranon physis and sclerosis compared to the normal contralateral side. A key point is that normal radiographs do not rule out an apophyseal injury. Some have used technetium Tc 99m bone scan to help confirm stress fractures.[2]

Initial treatment of olecranon apophysitis should be nonsurgical. Activity modification, NSAIDs, ice, and physical therapy usually help resolve symptoms by 4 to 6 weeks. If chronic apophysitis develops, surgical treatment may be warranted. Surgical treatment is indicated for patients with refractory symptoms and a documented failure of olecranon apophyseal closure after 3 to 6 months of nonsurgical treatment. Rudzki and Paletta[50] advocated using a single cancellous screw across the open apophysis for surgical fixation.

Figure 8 shows an olecranon apophyseal fracture treated with a cancellous screw. Postoperatively, the elbow should be immobilized for 10 days and then permitted only passive extension for 6 weeks.[50] At 6 weeks, active extension begins. At 8 weeks, the physical therapy regimen begins to incorporate gradual strengthening and range-of-motion exercises. Return to athletic activity can be estimated to take place at 3 months. Older patients with olecranon stress fractures should be treated similarly if nonsurgical treatment fails. Elbow arthroscopy can identify osteophytes or loose bodies that can subsequently be débrided. To compress the stress fracture, a 6.5- or 7.3-mm cannulated screw is placed down the intramedullary canal, crossing the fracture site or unfused apophysis.[5]

Posterior Compartment Injuries
As young athletes reach skeletal maturity, posteromedial impingement with osteophyte formation on the olecranon due to valgus extension overload syndrome may develop. Figure 2 demonstrates the location of osteophyte and symptom formation. In rare cases, the osteophytes fragment and become loose bodies.[5] Patients will report pain on terminal extension and on physical examination demonstrate a positive valgus extension overload test. In this test, the patient is seated and the shoulder rests in slight forward flexion. The examiner then forcefully extends the elbow while applying a valgus force. Pain with this maneuver usually indicates posteromedial impingement.[5] Additionally, UCL integrity should always be tested in elbows with posterior pain or decreased range of motion. Initial treatment involves rest and rehabilitation. Failure of nonsurgical treatment should lead one to attempt arthroscopic débridement.[5] The amount of olecranon osteophyte that can be excised without compromising elbow stability remains unknown. Usually, resecting just enough to allow full elbow extension (around 3 to 5 mm) suffices.[54]

Cubital Tunnel Syndrome
Ulnar neuritis can complicate medial-sided injuries such as medial apophysitis or UCL strain. However, ulnar neuropathy may also present on its own. Godshall and Hansen[55] first reported two cases of isolated ulnar neuropathy in 14-year-old Little League pitchers in 1971. Although only sporadically documented in the literature, the etiology is overuse during repetitive throwing. Patients report medial-sided elbow pain, often starting during periods of more intense throwing such as competitions. The pain returns even after a period of rest. Patients will also cite inability to extend the elbow without pain and weakness when grabbing balls. On physical examination, the athletes will have paresthesia in

the ulnar two fingers with static two-point discrimination >7 mm and pinch weakness. The elbow flexion test (passively flex elbow with forearm supination) exacerbates the paresthesias.[56] Medial valgus instability should be definitively ruled out by valgus stress-loading the elbow. Radiographs and MRI are often normal but sometimes show bone fragments medially or loose bodies. Electromyographic studies can help to confirm the diagnosis. Rest and NSAIDs represent the first-line therapy. When they fail to provide relief, a surgical ulnar nerve transposition can be attempted. Aoki and associates[57] performed an anterior subcutaneous transposition of the ulnar nerve on six adolescent baseball players with cubital tunnel syndrome. The nerve was completely released 7 cm proximal and 7 cm distal to the medial epicondyle. All patients had complete resolution of symptoms and return to throwing at 5 months postoperatively. After surgery, the arm was protected in a sling for 10 days. Then gentle, active range of motion was begun until the 4-week mark. Gentle throwing was started at 6 weeks.

PITCHING GUIDELINES

The USA Baseball Medical and Safety Advisory Committee has made several recommendations with the intent of preventing baseball injuries in skeletally immature athletes. The guidelines rely on a 1996 study commissioned by the Committee that interpreted survey responses.[58] Since then, recommendations have been updated based on more recent data.[59] The most recent Committee report (May 2006) advocates that children learn pitches no earlier than the following ages: fastball, age 8 years; change-up, age 10 years; curveball, age 14 years; knuckleball, age 15 years; and slider/forkball/split-ter/screwball, older than 16 years (**Table 2**). Furthermore, breaking pitches should not be taught until after skeletal maturity. Maximum pitch counts per game for various age groups are provided in **Table 3**. Pitchers should not compete more than 9 months a year and should avoid all overhead activities during the 3 months of rest. In general, a 9- to 14-year-old pitcher should have a limit of 75 competitive maximum effort pitches per game and a season limit of 1,000 pitches. In addition, a pitcher who experiences pain with throwing should be removed immediately, should never return to pitch the same day after being removed, and should not practice postgame competitive pitches. Pitchers younger than age 13 years should receive at least 3 days' rest after throwing more than four innings. Pitchers age 13 to 18 years require at least 3 days' rest after throwing more than five innings.

TABLE 2

Recommended Age for Learning Various Pitches

Pitch	Age (years)
Fastball	8 ± 2
Change-Up	10 ± 3
Curveball	14 ± 2
Knuckleball	15 ± 3
Slider	16 ± 2
Forkball	16 ± 2
Screwball	17 ± 2

Reproduced with permission from Andrews JR, Fleisig G: Medical and Safety Advisory Committee: Special Report. How many pitches should I allow my child to throw? *USA Baseball News* April 1996.

TABLE 3

Maximum Number of Pitches Recommended

Age (years)	Maximum Pitches/Game	Maximum Games/Week	Maximum Pitches/Week	Maximum Pitches/Season	Maximum Pitches/Year
8 to 10	50	2	75	1,000	2,000
11 to 12	75	2	100	1,000	3,000
13 to 14	75	2	125	1,000	3,000
15 to 16	90	2			
17 to 18	105	2			

Reproduced with permission from Andrews JR, Fleisig G: Medical and Safety Advisory Committee. Special Report: How many pitches should I allow my child to throw? *USA Baseball News* April 1996.

CONCLUSIONS

Management of elbow injuries in young athletes carries unique responsibilities, including knowledge of the developing elbow anatomy, sport-specific dangers, and, particularly in throwing athletes, careful evaluation of mechanics and training and performance volume. To mitigate elbow injuries in pediatric and adolescent athletes, guidelines to reduce overuse injuries should be applied and enforced as much as possible.

REFERENCES

1. Benjamin HJ, Briner WW Jr: Little league elbow. *Clin J Sport Med* 2005;15:37-40.

2. Ireland ML, Hutchinson MR: Upper extremity injuries in young athletes. *Clin Sports Med* 1995;14:533-569.

3. Do T, Herrera-Soto J: Elbow injuries in children. *Curr Opin Pediatr* 2003;15:68-73.

4. Morrey BF, Tanaka S, An KN: Valgus stability of the elbow: A definition of primary and secondary constraints. *Clin Orthop Relat Res* 1991;265:187-195.

5. Cain EL Jr, Dugas JR, Wolf RS, Andrews JR: Elbow injuries in throwing athletes: A current concepts review. *Am J Sports Med* 2003;31:621-635.

6. Ahmad CS, ElAttrache NS: Valgus extension overload syndrome and stress injury of the olecranon. *Clin Sports Med* 2004;23:665-676.

7. Andrews JR, Heggland EJ, Fleisig GS, Zheng N: Relationship of ulnar collateral ligament strain to amount of medial olecranon osteotomy. *Am J Sports Med* 2001;29:716-721.

8. Safran M, Ahmad CS, Elattrache NS: Ulnar collateral ligament of the elbow. *Arthroscopy* 2005;21:1381-1395.

9. Park MC, Ahmad CS: Dynamic contributions of the flexor-pronator mass to elbow valgus stability. *J Bone Joint Surg Am* 2004;86:2268-2274.

10. Kocher MS, Waters PM, Micheli LJ: Upper extremity injuries in the pediatric athlete. *Sports Med* 2000;30:117-135.

11. Fleisig GS, Andrews JR, Dillman CJ, Escamilla RF: Kinetics of baseball pitching with implications about injury mechanisms. *Am J Sports Med* 1995;23:233-239.

12. Wilson FD, Andrews JR, Blackburn TA, McCluskey G: Valgus extension overload in the pitching elbow. *Am J Sports Med* 1983;11:83-88.

13. Fleisig GS, Barrentine SW, Zheng N, Escamilla RF, Andrews JR: Kinematic and kinetic comparison of baseball pitching among various levels of development. *J Biomech* 1999;32:1371-1375.

14. Campbell KR, Hagood SS, Takagi Y, McFarland EG, Volk CP, Silberstein CE: Kinetic analysis of the elbow and shoulder in professional and little league pitchers. *Med Sci Sports Exerc* 1994;26:S175.

15. Voloshin I, Schena A: Elbow injuries, in Schepsis AA, Busconi BD (eds): *Sports Medicine*. Philadelphia, PA, Lippincott Williams & Wilkins, 2006.

16. Escamilla RF, Fleisig GS, Zheng N, Barrentine SW, Wilk KE, Andrews JR: Biomechanics of the knee during closed kinetic chain and open kinetic chain exercises. *Med Sci Sports Exerc* 1998;30:556-569.

17. Fleisig GS, Kingsley DS, Loftice JW, et al: Kinetic comparison among the fastball, curveball, change-up, and slider in collegiate baseball pitchers. *Am J Sports Med* 2006;34:423-430.

18. McFarland EG, Ireland ML: Rehabilitation programs and prevention strategies in adolescent throwing athletes. *Instr Course Lect* 2003;52:37-42.

19. Skaggs DL, Mirzayan R: The posterior fat pad sign in association with occult fracture of the elbow in children. *J Bone Joint Surg Am* 1999;81:1429-1433.

20. Miller TT, Adler RS, Friedman L: Sonography of injury of the ulnar collateral ligament of the elbow: Initial experience. *Skeletal Radiol* 2004;33:386-391.

21. Panner H: An affection of the capitulum humeri resembling Calve-Perthes disease of the hip. *Acta Radiol* 1927;8:617-618.

22. Douglas G, Rang M: The role of trauma in the pathogenesis of the osteochondroses. *Clin Orthop Relat Res* 1981;158:28-32.

23. Duthie RB, Houghton GR: Constitutional aspects of the osteochondroses. *Clin Orthop Relat Res* 1981;158:19-27.

24. Singer KM, Roy SP: Osteochondrosis of the humeral capitellum. *Am J Sports Med* 1984;12:351-360.

25. Yamaguchi K, Sweet FA, Bindra R, Morrey BF, Gelberman RH: The extraosseous and intraosseous arterial anatomy of the adult elbow. *J Bone Joint Surg Am* 1997;79:1653-1662.

26. Kobayashi K, Burton KJ, Rodner C, Smith B, Caputo AE: Lateral compression injuries in the pediatric elbow: Panner's disease and osteochondritis dissecans of the capitellum. *J Am Acad Orthop Surg* 2004;12:246-254.

27. Ruch DS, Poehling GG: Arthroscopic treatment of Panner's disease. *Clin Sports Med* 1991;10:629-636.

28. Lord J, Winell JJ: Overuse injuries in pediatric athletes. *Curr Opin Pediatr* 2004;16:47-50.

29. Lyman S, Fleisig GS, Waterbor JW, et al: Longitudinal study of elbow and shoulder pain in youth baseball pitchers. *Med Sci Sports Exerc* 2001;33:1803-1810.

30. Caine D, Howe W, Ross W, Bergman G: Does repetitive physical loading inhibit radial growth in female gymnasts? *Clin J Sport Med* 1997;7:302-308.

31. Caine DJ, Nassar L: Gymnastics injuries. *Med Sport Sci* 2005;48:18-58.

32. Fa K, E B, U H: Are bone bruises a possible cause of osteochondritis dissecans of the capitellum? A case report and review of the literature. *Arch Orthop Trauma Surg* 2005;125:545-549.

33. Griffith JF, Roebuck DJ, Cheng JC, et al: Acute elbow trauma in children: Spectrum of injury revealed by MR imaging not apparent on radiographs. *AJR Am J Roentgenol* 2001;176:53-60.

34. Petrie RBJ: Osteochondritis dissecans of the humeral capitellum, in De Lee JC, Drez D, Miller MD (eds): *Orthopaedic Sports Medicine: Principles and Practice.* Philadelphia, PA, WB Saunders, 2003.

35. Bradley J, Dandy DJ: Results of drilling osteochondritis dissecans before skeletal maturity. *J Bone Joint Surg Br* 1989;71:642-644.

36. Iwasaki N, Kato H, Ishikawa J, Saitoh S, Minami A: Autologous osteochondral mosaicplasty for capitellar osteochondritis dissecans in teenaged patients. *Am J Sports Med* 2006;34:1233-1239.

37. Kiyoshige Y, Takagi M, Yuasa K, Hamasaki M: Closed-wedge osteotomy for osteochondritis dissecans of the capitellum: A 7- to 12-year follow-up. *Am J Sports Med* 2000;28:534-537.

38. Yoshizu T: Closed wedge osteotomy for osteochondritis dissecans of humeral capitellus. *Orthopaedics (Seikeigeka)* 1986;37:1232-1242.

39. Bauer M, Jonsson K, Josefsson PO, Linden B: Osteochondritis dissecans of the elbow: A long-term follow-up study. *Clin Orthop Relat Res* 1992;284:156-160.

40. Hogan KA, Gross RH: Overuse injuries in pediatric athletes. *Orthop Clin North Am* 2003;34:405-415.

41. Chen FS, Diaz VA, Loebenberg M, Rosen JE: Shoulder and elbow injuries in the skeletally immature athlete. *J Am Acad Orthop Surg* 2005;13:172-185.

42. Hang DW, Chao CM, Hang YS: A clinical and roentgenographic study of Little League elbow. *Am J Sports Med* 2004;32:79-84.

43. Faigenbaum AD: Strength training for children and adolescents. *Clin Sports Med* 2000;19:593-619.

44. Farsetti P, Potenza V, Caterini R, Ippolito E: Long-term results of treatment of fractures of the medial humeral epicondyle in children. *J Bone Joint Surg Am* 2001;83:1299-1305.

45. Bede WB, Lefebvre AR, Rosman MA: Fractures of the medial humeral epicondyle in children. *Can J Surg* 1975;18:137-142.

46. Ireland ML, Andrews JR: Shoulder and elbow injuries in the young athlete. *Clin Sports Med* 1988;7:473-494.

47. Case SL, Hennrikus WL: Surgical treatment of displaced medial epicondyle fractures in adolescent athletes. *Am J Sports Med* 1997;25:682-686.

48. O'Driscoll SW, Lawton RL, Smith AM: The "moving valgus stress test" for medial collateral ligament tears of the elbow. *Am J Sports Med* 2005;33:231-239.

49. Barnes DA, Tullos HS: An analysis of 100 symptomatic baseball players. *Am J Sports Med* 1978;6:62-67.

50. Rudzki JR, Paletta GA Jr: Juvenile and adolescent elbow injuries in sports. *Clin Sports Med* 2004;23:581-608.

51. Argo D, Trenhaile SW, Savoie FH III, Field LD: Operative treatment of ulnar collateral ligament insufficiency of the elbow in female athletes. *Am J Sports Med* 2006;34:431-437.

52. Petty DH, Andrews JR, Fleisig GS, Cain EL: Ulnar collateral ligament reconstruction in high school baseball players: Clinical results and injury risk factors. *Am J Sports Med* 2004;32:1158-1164.

53. Gore RM, Rogers LF, Bowerman J, Suker J, Compere CL: Osseous manifestations of elbow stress associated with sports activities. *AJR Am J Roetgenol* 1980;134:971-977.

54. Reddy AS, Kvitne RS, Yocum LA, Elattrache NS, Glousman RE, Jobe FW: Arthroscopy of the elbow: A long-term clinical review. *Arthroscopy* 2000;16:588-594.

55. Godshall RW, Hansen CA: Traumatic ulnar neuropathy in adolescent baseball pitchers. *J Bone Joint Surg Am* 1971;53:359-361.

56. Tomaino MM, Brach PJ, Vansickle DP: The rationale for and efficacy of surgical intervention for electrodiagnostic-negative cubital tunnel syndrome. *J Hand Surg [Am]* 2001;26:1077-1081.

57. Aoki M, Kanaya K, Aiki H, Wada T, Yamashita T, Ogiwara N: Cubital tunnel syndrome in adolescent baseball players: A report of six cases with 3- to 5-year follow-up. *Arthroscopy* 2005;21:758.

58. Andrews J, Fleisig G: Medical and Safety Advisory Committee: Special Report. How many pitches should I allow my child to throw? *USA Baseball News* April 1996.

59. Lyman S, Fleisig GS, Andrews JR, Osinski ED: Effect of pitch type, pitch count, and pitching mechanics on risk of elbow and shoulder pain in youth baseball pitchers. *Am J Sports Med* 2002;30:463-468.

CHAPTER 2

LATERAL EPICONDYLITIS

JONATHAN D. PACKER, MD
DUONG NGUYEN, MD, FRCSC
MATTHEW A. KIPPE, MD
THEODORE A. BLAINE, MD

"Tennis elbow" (lateral epicondylitis) was first described by Runge[1] in 1873 as lateral elbow pain found in tennis players. However, 95% of all cases are seen in nonathletes,[2] with an annual incidence believed to be between 1% and 3% in the general population.[3-5] It is estimated that between 10% and 50% of people who regularly play tennis will have lateral epicondylitis at some point in their tennis careers.[6,7] The peak incidence is between the ages of 35 and 54 years,[3-5] and the prevalence rates in men and women are equal.[8] Most episodes of lateral epicondylitis last from 6 months to 2 years.[9]

The etiology of lateral epicondylitis is related to overuse of the wrist extensor muscles through repetitive motions. Movements in which the elbow is flexed while an object (like a racquet) is tightly gripped and activities that require pronation and supination with the elbow near full extension are frequent causes of lateral epicondylitis.[2] This type of movement places a high tension load on the wrist extensor muscles, especially the extensor carpi radialis brevis (ECRB). Common occupational causes of lateral epicondylitis include plumbing, painting, raking, weaving, gardening, and meat-cutting.

Tennis, racquetball, squash, and fencing are frequent causes among athletes.[10] The physiologic age of the tendon seems to be more important than the chronologic age.[11] Bernhang and associates[12] showed that more experienced players were found to have a decreased incidence as compared to novice players, despite more frequent play. This is because advanced players had a shorter duration of maximum grip pressure. Abnormal techniques include leading with a flexed elbow on backhand shots, incorrect positioning of the arm at ball strike, and striking the ball off the "sweet spot" of the racquet. Additionally, certain features are thought to increase the incidence of lateral epicondylitis, eg, decreased racquet stiffness, smaller sweet spots, harder playing surfaces, and high-tension strings. These factors place increased force loads on the upper extremity, particularly the wrist extensors. Repetitive overuse of the wrist extensors from nonathletic activities follows the same principle.

ANATOMY

The primary ECRB origin is located on the anterior aspect of the lateral epicondyle, lying deep and distal to the extensor carpi radialis longus (ECRL). The tendon also originates from the distal lateral humeral supracondylar ridge, the underside of the anterior medial edge of the extensor aponeurosis, the undersurface of the ECRL, the distal extensor aponeurosis, and the annular ligament.[13]

The relationships between the ECRB origin and the lateral collateral ligament, the annular ligament, and the radial nerve are important anatomic considerations. The lateral ulnar collateral ligament is the chief lateral stabilizer of the elbow.[14] The origins of the lateral collateral ligament, ECRB, and extensor digitorum communis (EDC) tendons are confluent and form a common tendinous origin. This common extensor origin was found to be a separate structure from that of the ECRL and extensor carpi ulnaris. The common extensor origin is in close proximity to the joint capsule, but there does not appear to be any interdigitation of the tendon with the capsule.[15]

TABLE 1	
Baker Arthroscopic Classification System for Capsular Pathology[21-23]	
Type I	Smooth capsule without irregularity; inflammation and fraying deep to the ECRB origin without evidence of frank tear
Type II	Linear or longitudinal tears at the under surface of the ECRB origin
Type III	Retracted with partial or complete avulsions of the tendon

Adapted with permission from Baker CL Jr, Jones GL: Arthroscopy of the elbow. *Am J Sports Med* 1999;27:251-264.

The radial nerve travels along the posterior humeral shaft. It penetrates the lateral intermuscular septum and descends anterior to the lateral epicondyle. After passing between the brachioradialis and brachialis muscles, the radial nerve branches to form the superficial radial nerve and the posterior interosseous nerve (PIN). The nerve can be injured during arthroscopic débridement directly anterior to the radial head.

In a cadaveric study, the annular ligament was found to have three layers.[16] The outermost layer is derived from the lateral ligament of the elbow. The middle layer is the annular band that attaches anteriorly to the radial notch of the ulna and posteriorly to the posterior margin of the radial notch. The innermost layer is formed by the joint capsule, which is continuous superiorly with the capsule of the elbow.

PATHOPHYSIOLOGY

There is increasing evidence that the etiology of lateral epicondylitis is multifactorial. Since 1936, the cause of lateral epicondylitis has been described as microscopic or macroscopic tears of the wrist extensor tendon origin with associated granulation tissue.[2,17-19] Nirschl and Pettrone[19] coined the term angiofibroblastic hyperplasia to describe this histologic abnormality, which is a disruption of the normal parallel arrangement of the tendon fibers by invasion of fibroblasts and vascular, atypical, granulation-like tissue. Many studies have suggested that lateral epicondylitis is more likely to be a degenerative process than an inflammatory process, although this supposition has not been confirmed. This process primarily involves the ECRB, with secondary involvement of the EDC.[11]

Recent studies suggest that a component of the pathology may also involve the joint capsule. Duparc and associates[20] described a synovial fold within the radiocapitellar joint as being responsible for lateral epicondylalgia of the elbow. Furthermore, Baker and associates[21] found a 69% incidence of capsular injury in patients with lateral epicondylitis undergoing arthroscopic treatment. The associated disorders included synovial pathology, bone spurs, valgus extension overload, loose bodies, and degenerative joint disease. Baker and associates[21-23] also described three distinct patterns of pathologic changes in the lateral joint capsule (**Table 1**). Type I lesions have inflammation and fraying deep to the ECRB tendon without evidence of a frank tear. Type II lesions are linear, or longitudinal, capsular tears. Type III lesions represent complete rupture and retraction of the capsule and the frayed ECRB tendon. Although this classification can be useful in describing pathologic changes within the joint, it has not been found to have any prognostic value in predicting outcome.

Mullett and associates[24] found a high incidence of radiocapitellar synovial hypertrophy in patients with lateral epicondylitis. They proposed that a degenerative capsulosynovial fold of the annular ligament impinges on the radial head and interposes in the anterior or posterior portions of the radiocapitellar joint. Compression of this tissue by contraction of the wrist extensors reproduced typical symptoms of lateral epicondylitis. Histologic analysis showed evidence of hyaline degeneration and subsynovial fibrosis, further supporting the degenerative hypothesis. Nerve fibers have been observed in this deep part of the synovial fold, offering a possible explanation for pain at rest despite the absence of inflammation.[20,24,25] Additionally, tendinosis of the ECRB origin can involve the lateral collateral ligament, a major stabilizer of the elbow.[14,26]

CLINICAL EVALUATION
History and Physical Examination
Occasionally a patient will recall a specific injury, but usually the onset is gradual and insidious. The patient reports discomfort over the lateral epicondyle that often

radiates down the dorsal forearm. The pain is exacerbated by lifting, gripping, or repetitive wrist activity. Patients may notice a loss of grip strength as well.

On physical examination, a palpable tenderness is localized slightly distal and anterior to the lateral epicondyle and extensor tendon, particularly in the early stages. Findings suggestive of lateral epicondylitis are pain near the lateral epicondyle with resistance to wrist extension or maximal wrist flexion with the elbow in full extension. Pain with resisted middle finger extension is diagnostic of ECRB tendinosis, whereas pain with resisted index finger extension is indicative of ECRL pathology. Discomfort with gripping is commonly found in the same region. Additionally, loss of wrist extension and grip strength compared to the unaffected side may be present.

Physicians should be aware of conditions that mimic elbow tendinosis such as cervical radiculopathy, radial tunnel syndrome, radial head fracture, radiocapitellar arthrosis, posterolateral rotatory instability, lateral synovial fringe, loose bodies, osteochondritis, and posterolateral impingement.[27] These causes of lateral elbow pain should be excluded with a thorough history and physical examination. Radial tunnel syndrome, which is present in up to 5% of patients with lateral epicondylitis,[28] can be differentiated by testing resisted supination.

Imaging Studies

Radiologic evaluation can be useful in ruling out other pathology. AP and lateral views of the elbow are typically ordered; frequently they show normal results. If nerve compression syndromes are suspected, cervical spine radiographs and electrodiagnostic studies may be necessary. MRI with gadolinium can aid in distinguishing between lateral epicondylitis, lateral collateral ligament tears, and avulsion of the common extensor tendon. False-positive MRI findings suggesting lateral collateral ligament tear are common and should be interpreted with reference to clinical examination findings. With degenerative tendinosis, there is increased signal intensity on T1-weighted images that is not as bright as fluid on T2-weighted images, as well as an increased thickness of the ECRB tendon. In the presence of a partial ECRB tear, tendon thinning can be seen, along with focal hyperintense signal involving a portion of the tendon on T2-weighted images.[29] Potter and associates[30] reported that the tendon degeneration and degree of the tear, as depicted on MRI,

correlated well with surgical and histologic findings. Also, in lateral epicondylitis, radiographic signs of calcification of soft tissue adjacent to the epicondyle have been reported in 7% to 25% of cases.[19,31]

NONSURGICAL TREATMENT

Initial treatment consists of rest, ice, nonsteroidal anti-inflammatory drugs (NSAIDs), and activity modification. In the acute phase, physical therapy modalities such as friction massage, manipulation, and stretching can be helpful in decreasing symptoms. After symptoms improve, a strengthening program for the extensor muscles is added. Bracing can be another useful adjunct.[32] Counterforce or wrist extension braces are thought to work by decreasing the load of the ECRB and EDC during contraction. This has corresponded to decreased extensor muscle activity demonstrated by electromyographic activity.[33] Iontophoresis of dexamethasone sodium phosphate has been shown to be effective in reducing symptoms of epicondylitis at short-term follow-up.[34] The mechanism by which extracorporeal shock-wave therapy (ESWT) relieves the lateral elbow pain is poorly understood. Although two trials[35,36] reported significant improvement with ESWT, a recent meta-analysis[37] of nine randomized controlled trials found that ESWT provides no increased benefit in terms of pain and function compared to other treatments.

Corticosteroid injection (typically betamethasone with lidocaine) is a common treatment of lateral epicondylitis that is unresponsive to rest, physical therapy, activity modification, and NSAID treatment. Patients should be warned about an increase in pain the first 24 hours after injection.[38] The most commonly used technique is to inject anterior to the lateral epicondyle and deep to the ECRB tendon. Given the growing evidence that part of the pathology of lateral epicondylitis may be intra-articular,[20-22,24,26] the use of intra-articular injections has generated interest because of their ease of administration and lower risk of complications (PIN anesthesia, subcutaneous fat atrophy, tendinous damage and rupture) as compared to extra-articular injections. In a recent cadaveric study, we investigated the localization and accuracy of both injection techniques. We found that not only did intra-articular injections reach the ECRB origin in 88% of injections, but also they were more successful than extra-articular injections at reaching both components of the presumed pathology (ECRB and capsule). Additionally, PIN diffusion was present in 50% of the extra-articular injections as compared to 0% of the intra-articular injections.

A recent meta-analysis of 13 randomized controlled trials revealed that corticosteroid injections for refractory lateral epicondylitis were beneficial in the short term (<6 weeks), but not at intermediate (6 weeks to 6 months) or long-term (>6 months) follow-up.[39] High-quality studies were lacking, however, so there was insufficient evidence to draw any firm conclusions.

Modification of sports technique or equipment should be considered in high-level athletes when symptoms persist. For tennis players, improved techniques that shift the strain from the upper extremity to core musculature and lower extremities have been effective. Additionally, proper grip size,[11] lighter racquets, low-vibration frames, low string tensions, and playing on slower surfaces can also decrease the strain on the wrist extensors.

SURGICAL TREATMENT

Indications

Despite nonsurgical treatment, chronic symptoms develop in 5% to 10% of patients and eventually require surgical intervention.[2,19,25,40-42] Indications for surgery are persistent, debilitating pain that inhibits patients from participating in desired activities and pain that is refractory to nonsurgical management.

Techniques

Both open and arthroscopic techniques have been described, with the common goals of débriding the diseased tissue and release of the ECRB origin.

Open Release

The most commonly used technique is described by Nirschl and Ashman.[13] The focus is on the excision of the ECRB tendon attachment to the anteromedial aspect of the extensor aponeurosis and débridement of diseased or pain-producing tissue. The ECRB tendon is almost always involved, the anterior edge of the EDC tendon is involved in half the cases, and occasionally the underside of the ECRL is involved.

In most cases, it is not necessary to reattach the remaining, healthy tendon to the surrounding tissue or bone.[13] The cortex of the lateral condylar triangular recess is drilled to create vascular channels and stimulate healing of healthy tissue. The lateral epicondyle is not altered, and the ECRL and EDC are anatomically repaired. Typically, the joint is not addressed unless there is clear clinical or radiographic evidence suggestive of intra-articular pathology.

The Nirschl mini-open surgical technique was first described in 1979.[19] With the patient in the supine position, several towels are placed under the elbow to internally rotate the shoulder. A small incision is made over the lateral aspect of the elbow, beginning just proximal to the lateral epicondyle and ending just distal to the radiocapitellar joint (**Figure 1**, *A*). The ECRL and extensor aponeurosis interface is identified and split to a depth of 2 to 3 mm (**Figure 1**, *B*). This interface can be found at the posterior region of the muscle belly of the ECRL. The goal is to lift the ECRL off the underlying ECRB without altering the ECRB. Retraction of the ECRL anteromedially brings the ECRB tendon into view as it attaches to the EDC aponeurosis. If rupture of the common extensor tendon is seen, it should be repaired with drill holes or suture anchors. Diseased tissue, which appears dull, gray, and friable, is identified and removed. Occasionally, the superficial fibers of the ECRB tendon appear normal and cover the diseased tissue. Diseased tissue can be grossly differentiated from healthy, shiny white tissue by its dull gray, bleeding appearance (**Figure 1**, *C*). The scratch test described by Nirschl and Ashman[13] can be used if identifying diseased tissue is difficult. A broad blade is used to scrape the suspect tissue, which will peel away if diseased. When an exostosis requires removal, the anterior aspect of the extensor aponeurosis is minimally reflected off the anteromedial aspect of the lateral epicondyle and the exostosis is removed by rongeur dissection. The skin incision is expanded 0.5 cm distally to access suspected intra-articular pathology such as loose bodies, synovitis, annular ligament infolding, valgus extension overload, and degenerative joint disease. A small longitudinal opening is made in the synovium anterior to the radial collateral ligament, and the lateral compartment is inspected. During final repair, the ECRL is firmly sutured to the anteromedial margin of the EDC aponeurosis with a running side-to-side suture. Postoperatively, the patient's elbow and wrist are typically immobilized for 48 hours, followed by range-of-motion exercises.

Advantages of the Nirschl mini-open surgical technique include clear visualization and access to the pathologic area; the diseased tissue can be removed in its

FIGURE 1

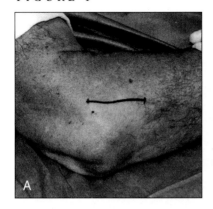 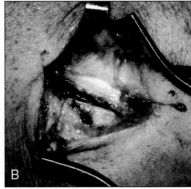 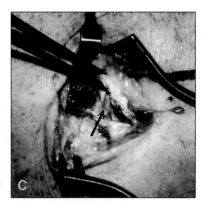

The Nirschl mini-open technique. **A,** The skin incision, beginning just proximal to the lateral epicondyle and ending just distal to the radiocapitellar joint, is marked. **B,** The ECRL and extensor aponeurosis interface is split. **C,** The diseased tissue (arrow) is identified.

entirety and the underlying bone decorticated. Disadvantages include violation of the extensor aponeurosis and the inability to address intra-articular pathology. Nirschl and Pettrone[19] reported 85% good or excellent results in 88 patients with this technique.

Percutaneous Release

The percutaneous release was first described by Yerger and Turner in 1985.[43] It is an office procedure that has reduced morbidity compared to the open release, but disadvantages include the possibility of an inadequate resection or recurrence. Unlike the open and arthroscopic releases, the diseased tissue is not removed in percutaneous release.[44] The patient's arm is sterilely prepared and draped. The periepicondylar area is anesthetized with a local anesthetic. A 1- to 2-cm incision is made transversely, anterior to the tip of the epicondyle. The common extensor tendon is then incised just distal to the lateral epicondyle. The surgeon's thumb is kept over the posterolateral aspect of the radiocapitellar joint to prevent extension of the scalpel and injury to the lateral ulnar collateral ligament.

Arthroscopic Release

The technique of arthroscopic treatment of lateral epicondylitis was first described in 1995 by Grifka and associates.[45] This approach provides excellent visualization of the joint, allows access to the pathologic lesion, and avoids dissection of the overlying healthy tissue. Arthroscopy also allows for assessment of intra-articular pathology, such as synovitis and loose bodies, and the ability to view

FIGURE 2

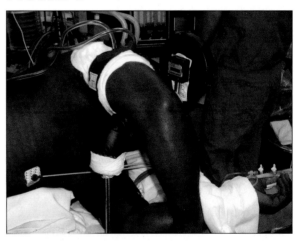

Patient in lateral decubitus position with arm in arm holder and nonsterile tourniquet applied. (Courtesy of William N. Levine, MD.)

the posterior compartment. The arthroscopic release involves excision of the diseased tissue with ECRB release and lateral epicondyle decortication with no repair of the ECRB defect.[21,22,46,47]

Patients are typically positioned in the lateral decubitus position with an arm holder (**Figure 2**), but the procedure can also be performed with the patient in the prone position. The joint is distended with 30 mL of fluid through an 18-gauge needle introduced through the lateral portal. This displaces the neurovascular structures anteriorly[46] and provides a more controlled entry into the joint with the arthro-

FIGURE 3

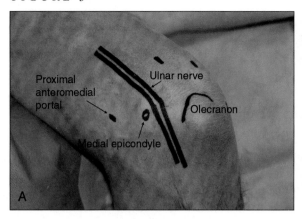 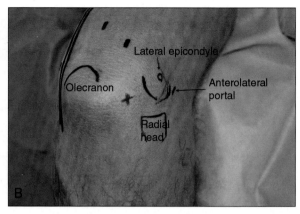

Anatomic landmarks are demonstrated in preparation for elbow arthroscopy. **A,** The olecranon tip, ulnar nerve, and medial epicondyle are marked on a right elbow. The proximal anteromedial portal is proximal and anterior to the medial epicondyle and is used for the 30° arthroscope to visualize the radiocapitellar joint for arthroscopic ECRB release. **B,** The olecranon tip and lateral epicondyle are marked. The anterolateral portal is anterior and proximal to the lateral epicondyle. The PIN is at risk if the portal is positioned too far distal. The anterolateral portal is used for débridement of the ECRB and capsule in arthroscopic ECRB release. (Courtesy of William N. Levine, MD.)

FIGURE 4

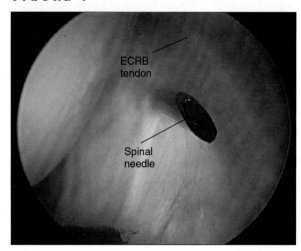

Arthroscopic view of the radiocapitellar joint from the proximal anteromedial portal. A spinal needle is introduced at the ECRB origin to localize the anterolateral portal placement.

scope. The standard viewing portal is the proximal anteromedial portal, which is located 2 cm proximal to the medial epicondyle and 1 cm anterior to the intermuscular septum, through a 30° scope (**Figure 3**). The joint should be inspected and any intra-articular pathology noted and addressed (**Figure 4**).

The capsule is inspected for any associated pathology and then resected to visualize the ECRB (**Figure 5**).

Beginning at its most proximal attachment, the tendon is released from the lateral epicondyle with the full radius resector (**Figure 6,** *A*) and then released from the condylar attachment to the radial head (**Figure 6,** *B*). Care should be taken to avoid damaging the articular surface and the lateral ulnar collateral ligament. The release of the ECRB tendon begins at the site of pathology and is followed back to the origin on the lateral epicondyle. To avoid injury to the lateral collateral ligament, the release should remain anterior to the bisector of the radial head with the elbow in 90° of flexion.[46] After release, a 4.5-mm round burr may be used to decorticate the lateral epicondyle and distal portion of the lateral condylar ridge in the area of the ECRB origin, although the need for decortication has recently been challenged. In one cadaveric study, Smith and associates[48] were able to resect the ECRB and EDC origins via standard arthroscopic techniques a mean of 100% and 90%, respectively. They concluded that complete resection of the common extensor (ECRB and EDC) origin is achievable while maintaining elbow stability.

Results

Several reports in the literature demonstrate the success of surgical treatment of lateral epicondylitis.

In a case series of 12 patients having arthroscopic ECRB release, the average return to unrestricted work following arthroscopy was 6 days.[47] None of these

FIGURE 5

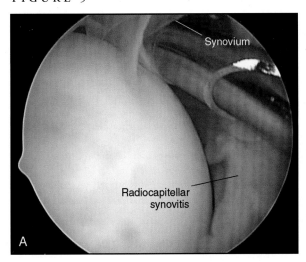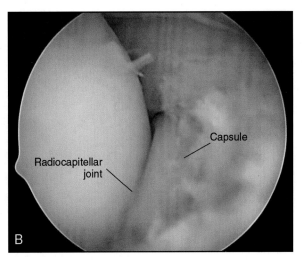

A, Arthroscopic view of the radiocapitellar joint from the proximal anteromedial portal. Radiocapitellar synovitis is seen and is débrided with the arthroscopic shaver. **B,** Arthroscopic view following débridement.

FIGURE 6

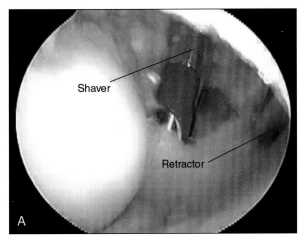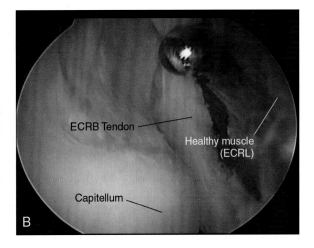

Arthroscopic views of the radiocapitellar joint from the proximal anteromedial portal. **A,** A retractor is used to improve visualization of the capsule and ECRB origin, and also helps to tension the tissue to facilitate débridement. **B,** The capsule is débrided with the shaver, followed by débridement of the ECRB tendon origin. Healthy muscle should be visualized following débridement.

patients experienced lateral instability from release of the lateral collateral ligament.[46,49] In another series of 42 arthroscopic releases,[21] associated intra-articular pathology was found in 69% of elbows at the time of arthroscopy. Thirty-seven of the 39 patients (95%) available for follow-up reported that they were "much better" or "better" after arthroscopic release. In another series, 17 of 20 patients (85%) reported a significant improvement after arthroscopic treatment.[50]

In two studies comparing open to arthroscopic release, the arthroscopic group returned to sports and work more quickly, but there was no difference in results between the two techniques.[51,52] In a trial comparing open and percutaneous releases, the percutaneous group had a significantly better subjective outcome, better basic Disabilities of the Arm, Shoulder and Hand (DASH) scores, and a quicker return to work.[53] In a recent retrospective study comparing percutaneous release with arthroscopic or open release, all three surgical methods resulted in a statistically significant improvement in postoperative Andrews-Carson scores, but there was no difference among the three groups.[54]

CONCLUSIONS

Nonsurgical treatment modalities for lateral epicondylitis are successful in most patients. When nonsurgical treatment fails, surgical treatment is a successful alternative. Open, arthroscopic, and percutanous release have all been shown to be successful and return patients to their desired activity level. Arthroscopic release may be associated with less morbidity and faster return to work. However, the surgical technique chosen should be tailored to the individual patient and surgeon experience.

REFERENCES

1. Runge F: Zur Genese und Behandlung des Schreibekrampfes. *Berliner Klin Wochenschr* 1873;10:245-248.

2. Coonrad RW, Hooper WR: Tennis elbow: Its course, natural history, conservative and surgical management. *J Bone Joint Surg Am* 1973;55:1177-1182.

3. Allander E: Prevalence, incidence, and remission rates of some common rheumatic diseases or syndromes. *Scand J Rheumatol* 1974;3:145-153.

4. Chard MD, Hazleman BL: Tennis elbow: A reappraisal. *Br J Rheumatol* 1989;28:186-190.

5. Chop WM Jr: Tennis elbow. *Postgrad Med* 1989;86:301-304.

6. Allman FL: Tennis elbow: Etiology, prevention and treatment. *Clin Orthop Relat Res* 1975;3:308-316.

7. Nirschl RP: Tennis elbow. *Orthop Clin North Am* 1973;4:787-800.

8. Gruchow HW, Pelletier D: An epidemiologic study of tennis elbow: Incidence, recurrence, and effectiveness of prevention strategies. *Am J Sports Med* 1979;7:234-238.

9. Murtagh JE: Tennis elbow. *Aust Fam Physician* 1988;17:90-91.

10. Jobe FW, Ciccotti MG: Lateral and medial epicondylitis of the elbow. J Am Acad Orthop Surg 1994;2:1-8.

11. Nirschl RP: Elbow tendinosis/tennis elbow. *Clin Sports Med* 1992;11:851-870.

12. Bernhang AM, Dehner W, Fogarty C: Tennis elbow: A biomechanical approach. *J Sports Med* 1974;2:235-260.

13. Nirschl RP, Ashman ES: Tennis elbow tendinosis (epicondylitis). *Instr Course Lect* 2004;53:587-598.

14. Cohen MS, Hastings H II: Rotatory instability of the elbow: The anatomy and role of the lateral stabilizers. *J Bone Joint Surg Am* 1997;79:225-233.

15. Greenbaum B, Itamura J, Vangsness CT, Tibone J, Atkinson R: Extensor carpi radialis brevis: An anatomical analysis of its origin. *J Bone Joint Surg Br* 1999;81:926-929.

16. Martin BF: The annular ligament of the superior radioulnar joint. *J Anat* 1958;92:473-482.

17. Cyriax JH: The pathology and treatment of tennis elbow. *J Bone Joint Surg Am* 1936;18:921-940.

18. Goldie I: Epicondylitis lateralis humeri (epicondylalgia or tennis elbow): A pathogenetical study. *Acta Chir Scand* Suppl. 1964;57:1.

19. Nirschl RP, Pettrone FA: Tennis elbow: The surgical treatment of lateral epicondylitis. *J Bone Joint Surg Am* 1979;61:832-839.

20. Duparc F, Putz R, Michot C, Muller JM, Freger P: The synovial fold of the humeroradial joint: Anatomical and histological features, and clinical relevance in lateral epicondylalgia of the elbow. *Surg Radiol Anat* 2002;24:302-307.

21. Baker CL Jr, Murphy KP, Gottlob CA, Curd DT: Arthroscopic classification and treatment of lateral epicondylitis: Two-year clinical results. *J Shoulder Elbow Surg* 2000;9:475-482.

22. Baker CL Jr, Jones GL: Arthroscopy of the elbow. *Am J Sports Med* 1999;27:251-264.

23. Baker CL, Cummings PD: Arthroscopic management of miscellaneous elbow disorders. *Oper Tech Sports Med* 1998;6:16-21.

24. Mullett H, Sprague M, Brown G, Hausman M: Arthroscopic treatment of lateral epicondylitis: Clinical and cadaveric studies. *Clin Orthop Relat Res* 2005;439:123-128.

25. Boyer MI, Hastings H: Lateral tennis elbow: Is there any science out there? *J Shoulder Elbow Surg* 1999;8:481-491.

26. Kalainov DM, Cohen MS: Posterolateral rotatory instability of the elbow in association with lateral epicondylitis. A report of three cases. *J Bone Joint Surg Am* 2005;87:1120-1125.

27. Dlabach JA, Baker CL: Lateral and medial epicondylitis in the overhead athlete. *Oper Tech Orthop* 2001;11:46-54.

28. Gabel GT, Morrey BF: Tennis elbow. *Instr Course Lect* 1998;47:165-172.

29. Banks KP, Ly JQ, Beall DP, Grayson DE, Bancroft LW, Tall MA: Overuse injuries of the upper extremity in the competitive athlete: Magnetic resonance imaging find-

ings associated with repetitive trauma. *Curr Probl Diagn Radiol* 2005;34:127-142.

30. Potter HG, Hannafin JA, Morwessel RM, DiCarlo EF, O'Brien SJ, Altchek DW: Lateral epicondylitis: Correlation of MR imaging, surgical, and histopathologic findings. *Radiology* 1995;196:43-46.

31. Pomerance J: Radiographic analysis of lateral epicondylitis. *J Shoulder Elbow Surg* 2002;11:156-157.

32. Froimson AI: Treatment of tennis elbow with forearm support band. *J Bone Joint Surg Am* 1971;53:183-184.

33. Groppel JL, Nirschl RP: A mechanical and electromyographical analysis of the effects of various joint counterforce braces on the tennis player. *Am J Sports Med* 1986;14:195-200.

34. Nirschl RP, Rodin DM, Ochiai DH, Maartmann-Moe C: Iontophoretic administration of dexamethasone sodium phosphate for acute epicondylitis: A randomized, double-blinded, placebo-controlled study. *Am J Sports Med* 2003;31:189-195.

35. Pettrone FA, McCall BR: Extracorporeal shock wave therapy without local anesthesia for chronic lateral epicondylitis. *J Bone Joint Surg Am* 2005;87:1297-1304.

36. Rompe JD, Theis C, Maffulli N: Shock wave treatment for tennis elbow [in German]. *Orthopade* 2005;34:567-570.

37. Buchbinder R, Green SE, Youd JM, Assendelft WJ, Barnsley L, Smidt N: Systematic review of the efficacy and safety of shock wave therapy for lateral elbow pain. *J Rheumatol* 2006;33:1351-1363.

38. Lewis M, Hay EM, Paterson SM, Croft P: Local steroid injections for tennis elbow: Does the pain get worse before it gets better? Results from a randomized controlled trial. *Clin J Pain* 2005;21:330-334.

39. Smidt N, Assendelft WJ, van der Windt DA, Hay EM, Buchbinder R, Bouter LM: Corticosteroid injections for lateral epicondylitis: A systematic review. *Pain* 2002;96:23-40.

40. Boyd HB, McLeod AC Jr: Tennis elbow. *J Bone Joint Surg Am* 1973;55:1183-1187.

41. Gardner RC: Tennis elbow: Diagnosis, pathology and treatment: Nine severe cases treated by a new recon-

structive operation. *Clin Orthop Relat Res* 1970;72:248-253.

42. Calvert PT, Allum RL, Macpherson IS, Bentley G: Simple lateral release in treatment of tennis elbow. *J R Soc Med* 1985;78:912-915.

43. Yerger B, Turner T: Percutaneous extensor tenotomy for chronic tennis elbow: An office procedure. *Orthopedics* 1985;8:1261-1263.

44. Organ SW, Nirschl RP, Kraushaar BS, Guidi EJ: Salvage surgery for lateral tennis elbow. *Am J Sports Med* 1997;25:746-750.

45. Grifka J, Boenke S, Kramer J: Endoscopic therapy in epicondylitis radialis humeri. *Arthroscopy* 1995;11:743-748.

46. Kuklo TR, Taylor KF, Murphy KP, Islinger RB, Heekin RD, Baker CL Jr: Arthroscopic release for lateral epicondylitis: A cadaveric model. *Arthroscopy* 1999;15:259-264.

47. Owens BD, Murphy KP, Kuklo TR: Arthroscopic release for lateral epicondylitis. *Arthroscopy* 2001;17:582-587.

48. Smith AM, Castle JA, Ruch DS: Arthroscopic resection of the common extensor origin: Anatomic considerations. *J Shoulder Elbow Surg* 2003;12:375-379.

49. Morrey BF: Acute and chronic instability of the elbow. *J Am Acad Orthop Surg* 1996;4:117-128.

50. Jerosch J, Schunck J: Arthroscopic treatment of lateral epicondylitis: Indication, technique and early results. *Knee Surg Sports Traumatol Arthrosc* 2006;14:379-382.

51. Stapleton T, Baker C: Arthroscopic treatment of lateral epicondylitis: A clinical study [abstract]. *Arthroscopy* 1996;12:365-366.

52. Cohen M, Romeo A: Lateral epicondylitis: Open and arthroscopic treatment. *J Am Soc Surg Hand* 2001;1:172-176.

53. Dunkow PD, Jatti M, Muddu BN: A comparison of open and percutaneous techniques in the surgical treatment of tennis elbow. *J Bone Joint Surg Br* 2004;86:701-704.

54. Szabo SJ, Savoie FH, Field LD, Ramsey JR, Hosemann CD: Tendinosis of the extensor carpi radialis brevis: An evaluation of three methods of operative treatment. *J Shoulder Elbow Surg* 2006;15:721-727.

CHAPTER *3*

TREATMENT OF DISTAL BICEPS INJURIES

WILLIAM N. LEVINE, MD
DANIEL E. PRINCE, MD, MPH

ANATOMY

The biceps muscle is the most superficial muscle of the anterior compartment of the arm. The other muscles of the anterior compartment are the brachialis, which lies laterally, and the coracobrachialis, which lies deep to the biceps and inserts proximal to the elbow. All three muscles are innervated by the musculocutaneous nerve except the lateral aspect of the brachialis, which is innervated by the radial nerve. The biceps is a bipennate muscle proximally, with the long head originating on the superior labrum and the short head originating on the coracoid process as the conjoint tendon.

MRI studies have shown that the biceps tendon is a flattened cord approximately 10 cm in length from the ventral surface of the biceps muscle to its insertion on the radial tuberosity.[1] The tendon rotates as it approaches its insertion so the ventral surface lies against the radius. The distal biceps tendon attachment is enhanced by the bicipital aponeurosis, which courses off the medial aspect of the musculotendinous junction after passing the antecubital fossa. The aponeurosis joins the fascia of the flexor tendon mass and inserts medially on the subcutaneous border of the ulna. Because of the distal insertion of the biceps onto the radial tuberosity, biceps contraction acts on the forearm in two ways—flexion and supination. Studies have shown that the biceps provides approximately 30% of flexion strength and 40% of supination strength.[2,3]

The blood supply to the biceps tendon is from two to four branches off the anterolateral surface of the brachial artery, which supplies the proximal third of the tendon, and from one to three branches off the posterior recur-rent artery, which supplies the distal third.[4] Between the two vascularized zones is a 2-cm zone that is relatively hypovascular; its arterial supply depends solely on the longitudinal plexus of vessels within the paratenon.[4]

EPIDEMIOLOGY/NATURAL HISTORY

Complete distal biceps tendon (DBT) ruptures in the general population are rare. Safran and Graham[5] recently reported an incidence of 1.24 spontaneous complete DBT ruptures per 100,000 people per year, using California's electronic database from 1994 to 1998. Traditionally, distal ruptures have been estimated to comprise 3% of all biceps tendon ruptures.[6-8] However, the true incidence of complete DBT ruptures may be underestimated because some patients may not have sought medical attention or were incorrectly diagnosed. The incidence of partial biceps tendon injuries is more difficult to predict, as it is even more susceptible to the same confounders.

DBT ruptures typically occur in men between 30 and 50 years of age. Only one complete DBT rupture and three partial ruptures have been reported in the literature in women. The complete rupture occurred in an 82-year-old woman who sustained an eccentric force to her outstretched hand while falling.[5] Rantanen and Orava[9] performed a meta-analysis of the literature of all cases of DBT ruptures and found that most were men. The average age of patients sustaining distal biceps ruptures is 45 years (range, 25 to 70).[9-12]

Although DBT injuries are associated with a traumatic inciting event, there is evidence implicating an underlying degenerative tendon in afflicted patients. Seiler and associates[4] proposed a 2-cm hypovascular zone both in the DBT and its surrounding paratenon, marking this as a potential transition area that may have limited ability for repair. They also showed with CT that pronation of the arm resulted in a decrease of 50% in the cross-sectional area available to the tendon, and they hypothesized that bony irregularities or inflammation in the tendon could cause further impingement of the tendon.[4] MRI studies of chronic bicipitoradial bursitis have shown fluid within the bursa between the anterior cortex of the radial tuberosity and the DBT.[13,14] This bursa serves to reduce friction between the two structures during movement. Chronic inflammation of the bursa may weaken the DBT, predisposing the tendon to rupture with an acute insult.

Furthermore, Safran and Graham[5] found that tobacco smoking was strongly associated with DBT ruptures. They attribute the anoxic effects of smoking to the susceptible hypovascular region of the biceps tendon leading to increased degeneration. A mechanism of decreased blood flow, tissue hypoxia, and repetitive mechanical damage at an area with a diminished potential to repair may result in fiber degeneration and permanent weakness of the tendon, predisposing it to rupture when an eccentric strain is applied. Biomechanical studies have shown that the tensile strength of tendons decreases with increasing age, a fact that sheds light on the correlation between the fifth decade of life and DBT ruptures.[15]

Traditionally, athletes (specifically weight lifters) and heavy laborers were believed to be at higher risk for DBT ruptures than the general population.[16] In their meta-analysis, Rantanen and Orava[9] found that when the injury mechanism was reported, 62% were work-related, 30% were sports-related, and only 8% were leisure-related. Bell and associates[11] found that the injury occurred at work in 57% of patients. However, Safran and Graham[5] found that only 29% of patients were heavy laborers or athletes. There is no clear consensus as to etiology, as athletes may be at higher risk for other reasons, including the use of anabolic steroids that are implicated as a risk factor for DBT rupture and participation in higher risk activities.

CLASSIFICATION

There is currently no classification described for DBT tears. Commonly, tears of the DBT are described both by the degree and chronicity of injury. Tears can be complete or partial and can be either acute or chronic. Because tendon retraction occurs in a relatively short period of time, several weeks may be sufficient to transform an acute tear into a chronic tear.

CLINICAL EVALUATION/ PRESENTATION

DBT ruptures commonly occur with an unexpected extension force applied to a partially flexed elbow, resulting in a sudden, sharp, painful tearing sensation in the antecubital fossa. Most patients report both pain and weakness of elbow flexion, which gradually resolves. Some patients report weakness or pain with supination. Ecchymosis over the distal biceps muscle or in the antecubital fossa may occur after the inciting event. Patients may also report an obvious difference in the contour of the arm in this region. After the acute event, many patients attempt to resume activity, but they struggle with pain and weakness, reporting a dull ache that lasts several weeks.[17,18]

A visible defect may be appreciated in the distal arm when compared with the contralateral side (**Figure 1**). This is accentuated with resisted flexion of the elbow, as the biceps muscle belly is retracted proximally; however, if the bicipital aponeurosis (lacertus fibrosus) is intact, this may be less noticeable. Physical examination may reveal a palpable defect in the DBT and tenderness over the distal biceps muscle or antecubital region.

Ruland and associates[19] recently described the "biceps squeeze test" for diagnosis of complete DBT rupture. They reported the test had a 96% sensitivity for complete tendon rupture and no false negatives. Furthermore, the test could be used reliably postoperatively to show the effectiveness of the surgical repair. Additionally, in patients who had symptoms consistent with a DBT rupture but a negative squeeze test, there was an association with a partial biceps tendon rupture diagnosed via surgery or MRI.

Partial DBT tears are difficult to diagnose because they do not present with classic signs and symptoms of complete ruptures; however, MRI has increased the ability to diagnose partial DBT tears.[20] Patients often complain only of vague pain in the antecubital fossa, while examination consistently shows tenderness to palpation over the distal tendon and weakness against resisted supination.[21-23] Vardakas and associates[21] reported on seven patients with partial DBT tears, of whom only two

FIGURE 1

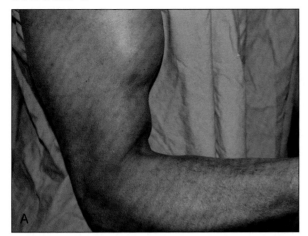 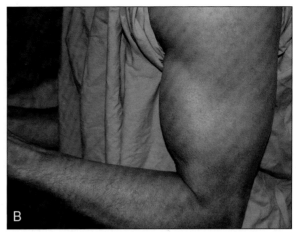

A 66-year-old right hand dominant man suffered an acute right biceps rupture doing pull-ups 3 weeks before presentation. Clinical photographs demonstrate **(A)** the "Popeye" deformity on the injured right arm and **(B)** the normal distal biceps contour on the left arm.

recalled an inciting event, while Dellaero and Mallon[23] reported on a series of seven patients with partial tears, of whom five recalled a specific inciting event. Kelly and associates[22] reported that half of the eight patients they studied recalled an inciting event. Prior to 2000, only six cases of partial biceps tendon tears were reported in the literature.[24-27] Since 2000, 27 additional cases have been reported, which is likely due to the increased diagnostic ability of MRI.[21-23,28,29]

IMAGING

Some authors believe that an accurate history and a confirmatory physical examination are sufficient to make a diagnosis without imaging studies.

Radiography

Radiographs of the elbow are usually normal; however, an avulsion fracture, hypertrophy, or irregularity of the radial tuberosity can be detected.

Magnetic Resonance Imaging

MRI for DBT ruptures is currently the gold standard to distinguish partial and complete tendon ruptures.[30,31] MRI is also helpful to diagnose intrasubstance tears and tears at the musculotendinous junction, as well as to determine if the bicipital aponeurosis is intact. Complete

rupture is characterized by absence of the tendon distally at its insertion site on the radial tuberosity on axial images. Retraction of the tendon can best be appreciated and measured on sagittal images. Partial tendon rupture is characterized by an increased signal within a thickened or thinned tendon, bone-marrow edema in the tuberosity, and fluid in the bicipitoradial bursa. Partial ruptures are difficult to distinguish from tendinopathy on MRI.

Recently, Giuffrè and Moss[1] described a novel positioning of the elbow for MRI in suspected cases of biceps tendon injury—shoulder abducted, elbow flexed, and forearm supinated. This allows the tendon to be seen in its entirety from origin to insertion on a single image, eliminating problems with partial volume-average effects. With the elbow flexed, the biceps contracts, pulling the tendon taut to its full length and allowing differentiation of partial and complete ruptures. It also allows improved visualization of the tendon nearest to the radial tuberosity, an area often difficult to evaluate with traditional positioning.

Ultrasonography

Recently, Miller and Adler[32] used ultrasonography with good results to diagnose both complete and partial tears of the DBT in seven patients. In patients with complete rupture, ultrasonography correctly identified four of five ruptures. The fifth patient was diagnosed with a partial rupture with retraction based on both ultrasonography and MRI, although at surgery 12 days later, the rupture was found to be complete. Ultrasonography diagnosed the other two patients with partial tendon ruptures; one was confirmed at surgery and the other underwent nonsurgical treatment with good results. The longitudinal axis is the best for showing tendon discontinuity and amount of retraction as both the tendon edge and radial tuberosity can be visualized simultaneously. Partial tears can be visualized on both axial and longitudinal images as thickening and altered echogeneity are seen. One advantage of ultrasonography over MRI is the ease of assessing the contralateral arm for comparison of bursal fluid, tendon retraction, tendon thickness, and underlying tendinopathy. Ultrasonography is operator-dependent, however, and with the infrequency of DBT ruptures, may be impractical. Larger, prospectively designed studies are necessary to determine the true cost-effectiveness of ultrasonography to replace MRI as the gold standard.

INDICATIONS

Because of the reproducibly good functional results of surgical treatment, repair of complete DBT injuries is indicated for all active and compliant patients. The resultant loss of flexion and supination strength and endurance without repair is marked, especially in the dominant arm, which is the more commonly injured arm. Nonsurgical treatment can be considered for the nondominant arm in low-demand patients older than 50 years of age.[33] Nonsurgical treatment consists of nonsteroidal anti-inflammatory drugs, splinting, and physical therapy.

Partial DBT tears can be initially treated nonsurgically. If the patient continues to have pain and weakness interfering with activities of daily living or physical demands, however, surgical exploration, detachment, and anatomic reattachment have been shown to decrease pain and return patients to their previous level of activity.[21-24,27]

Chronic ruptures of the DBT are not uncommon presentations for complete DBT tears because of delayed presentation by patients, the frequency of missed diagnosis, and the failure of nonsurgical management. Surgical repair of chronic tears is technically more difficult because the muscle and tendon retract proximally.[34] Recent studies of reconstructed chronic DBT tears have shown excellent results. Sanchez-Sotelo and associates[34]

reported on a case series of four patients who underwent surgery an average of 10.7 months (range, 3.6 to 18 months) after injury with an Achilles tendon allograft; all four had good or excellent outcomes. Hallam and Bain[35] reported on nine patients who underwent surgery an average of 4.1 months (range, 2.5 to 6.5) after injury with an autologous semitendinosus graft, with a postoperative mean Mayo elbow performance score of 96.3 (range, 85 to 100) and 100% patient satisfaction. Levy and associates[36] reported on five patients who underwent surgery at least 3 months after injury; they used half of the patient's flexor carpi radialis tendon with good postoperative results, including 100% patient satisfaction, full range of motion, and normal strength in flexion/extension. Because of the favorable published results for chronic DBT tears, reconstruction with augmentation of the retracted biceps tendon is indicated in patients with pain or weakness interfering with activities of daily living.

SURGICAL TREATMENT OPTIONS

Multiple surgical options are available for the repair of DBT ruptures: tenodesis to the brachialis muscle, anatomic reattachment via transosseous suture tunnel, and anatomic reattachment via suture anchors and/or interference screws. Additionally, the surgeon must decide between a two-incision technique and a single-incision technique for either of the anatomic reattachment options.

Klonz and associates[37] directly compared anatomic reattachment of complete DBT ruptures to tenodesis of the avulsed biceps tendon to the brachialis muscle in 14 patients. The authors found that anatomic repair restored an average strength of flexion of 96.8% (range, 78.9% to 113%) compared to 96% (range, 65.2% to 110.2%) for brachialis tenodesis. Power of supination was restored to 90.8% (range, 62.5% to 128.6%) for anatomic repair, but was only 76.6% (range, 42% to 150%) for brachialis tenodesis. There were four cases of heterotopic ossification in the anatomic reinsertion group, as well as two patients who reported pain in the antecubital fossa. One of these patients reported constant pain and paresthesia on the palmar radial forearm. After brachialis tenodesis, three patients reported anterior elbow pain, and one patient reported marked weakness of flexion and supination. One patient in each treatment group was dissatisfied—one after anatomic reinsertion, because of heterotopic ossification, pain, and mild sensory nerve damage; and the other after brachialis tenodesis, because of considerable weakness.[37] Bell and associates[11] reported a marked decrease of 16% in supination strength and an increase in flexion strength of 11% in their report of four patients treated with tenodesis to the brachialis.

SURGICAL TECHNIQUE

Acquaviva is credited with the first surgical reattachment of a ruptured DBT to the radial tuberosity in 1898.[38] In 1956, Fischer and Shepanek[39] described their technique for reattachment via a single anterior incision; however, Meherin and Kilgore[40] later reported on three patients who sustained permanent partial radial nerve injury with this technique. As a result, Boyd and Anderson[41] proposed a two-incision technique to eliminate potential damage to the radial nerve. Reports of radioulnar synostosis using the two-incision technique by Failla and associates[42] prompted a modified approach to decrease the incidence of synostosis. There has been renewed interest in the single-incision technique with the increasing versatility of suture anchors and interference screws.

Fixation

Traditionally, the DBT was reattached anatomically by tunneling into the radial tuberosity, grasping the distal tendon with a Krackow stitch, and tying the sutures down into the tunnel through transosseous suture holes. Alternatively, newer techniques use suture anchors into the radial tuberosity to anatomically restore the DBT.

Berlet and associates[43] compared the in vitro strength of bone tunnel fixation against two distinct single suture anchors, the Statak 5.2 mm (Zimmer, Warsaw, IN) and the Mitek G4 Superanchor (DePuy Mitek, Raynham, MA), in cadaveric models. This study showed that the yield strength of the bone tunnels was significantly higher than that of the single anchors, with no significant difference between the Statak and Mitek anchors (307 N versus 220 N and 187 N, respectively, $P < 0.05$). One limitation of the study was the use of four sutures in the bone tunnel technique compared to only two sutures in the anchor technique. This study also showed that under cyclic loading conditions,

none of the three fixation modalities failed. Other studies have supported the finding that single-suture anchor fixation has a lower yield strength compared to bone tunnel fixation.[44,45]

Lemos and associates[46] directly compared the use of two suture anchors to bone tunnels using the same number and size of suture material in cadaveric models. The suture anchor technique had a significantly higher yield strength compared to the bone tunnels (263 N versus 203 N, $P < 0.05$). Only one of nine suture anchors failed due to fixation, while five of nine bone tunnels failed due to breakage of the tunnels. Neither of the fixation techniques had an increased bone-tendon gap >1 cm at time of failure. This study is limited in that it measures only the tension force to failure and does not take into account cyclical loading of the fixation.

One Incision Versus Two Incisions

Assessing the outcomes of the single-incision technique compared to the two-incision technique is difficult because all studies use suture anchors in the single-incision technique and transosseous tunnels in the two-incision technique, confounding the outcomes due not only to the incision but also to the manner of fixation.

Sotereanos and associates[47] reported on the use of the single-incision technique in 16 patients using two 4.5-mm suture anchors with No. 2 nonabsorbable suture with good results. The average strength of flexion and supination was +10.9% and −5.3% postoperatively compared to the uninvolved side, respectively. The postoperative range of motion was excellent, with all patients experiencing full flexion, pronation, and supination, and an average decrease of only 0.6° (range, 0° to 10°). All 16 patients returned to their preinjury level of activity or employment and were satisfied with their outcomes.

El-Hawary and associates[48] compared 9 patients whose injuries were repaired anatomically via a single anterior incision with suture anchors to 10 patients whose injuries were repaired via two incisions with transosseous tunnels. There was increased elbow flexion motion in the single-incision technique compared to the two-incision technique (143° versus 131°), but there was no statistical difference in supination, pronation, or extension; strength of flexion or extension at 1 year; or functional outcome measured via the Short Form-36 scores. The authors reported a complication rate of 44% for the single-incision technique—three

FIGURE 2

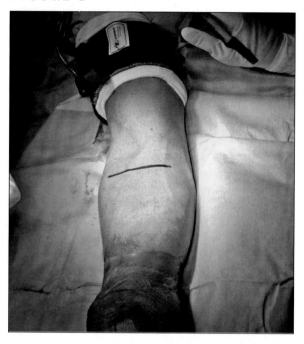

Right arm positioned on hand table in preparation for distal biceps repair.

cases of transient lateral antebrachial cutaneous nerve paresthesia, one flexion contracture, and one case of heterotopic ossification. The only complication reported with the two-incision technique was a transient superficial radial nerve paresthesia, resulting in a complication rate of 10%. Excluding the transient paresthesias, the complication rates for the single-incision and two-incision techniques decrease to 20% and 0%, respectively.

Bell and associates[11] reported on a series of 21 patients who underwent repair via the two-incision technique, but with one of three fixation techniques: transosseous tunnels (11 elbows), Mitek suture anchors (5 elbows), or screw fixation (5 elbows). They did not delineate the outcomes based on type of fixation, but reported an overall rate of heterotopic ossification of 61.9% (13 of 21 elbows) with the modified two-incision technique. There was no statistical difference between the type of fixation and the incidence of heterotopic ossification: Mitek anchors, 3 of 5; transosseous tunnels, 7 of 11; and screw fixation, 3 of 5. Complications in addition to the heterotopic ossification included one case of synostosis and one case of rupture of the tendon, both

occurring in transosseous tunnel repairs. The authors reported no infections, radial nerve injuries, or hardware failure.[11]

There is no prospectively designed study available to compare the single-incision and two-incision techniques for suture anchor fixation as to rates of nerve injury, heterotopic ossification, or failure of hardware. In vitro studies are encouraging for the use of two suture anchors via a single anterior approach to decrease the rates of heterotopic ossification while maintaining low risk to the radial nerve and adequate fixation.

Single-Incision and Two-Incision Techniques

Both techniques are highly successful when surgeons adhere to the principles outlined above. Although we perform both techniques, more often we perform the two-incision technique of Boyd and Anderson[41] popularized by Morrey. We have found it to be anatomically reproducible in restoring the biceps footprint, and by adhering to the surgical and anatomic principles highlighted by Morrey and others, we have avoided the complications that are detailed above.

Patient Positioning

For both single- and double-incision techniques, the patient is placed in the supine position with the arm on a hand table (**Figure 2**). All bony prominences are well padded to protect against intraoperative nerve compression or injury.

Incisions

The volar incision (the only incision for the single-incision technique) is made in the antecubital fossa to identify and retrieve the ruptured biceps tendon (**Figure 3**). The lateral antebrachial nerve is at risk in this incision, as is the basilic vein. Two running Krackow sutures are placed in the ruptured tendon to assist in mobilization and to secure the tendon. The second incision is made on the dorsal forearm, splitting the extensors and exposing the radial tuberosity.

Tendon Preparation

For single-incision techniques, a running Krackow suture and EndoButton (Smith and Nephew

Endoscopy, Andover, MA) are often used to incorporate the tendon (**Figure 4, A**). For the two-incision technique, two running Krackow sutures are placed so

there are four suture strands for later passage and suturing (**Figure 4, B**).

Radial Tuberosity Preparation

The radius is carefully exposed and baby Hohmann retractors are placed to ensure that no neurovascular structures are in harm's way. A 1-cm hole is then made in the anatomic footprint of the radial tuberosity with a Hall burr for tendon insertion (**Figure 5, A**).

If a single-incision approach is used, a technique using an EndoButton has been shown to be quite effective. A 4.5-mm drill is used to penetrate the far cortex (**Figure 5, B**) and then a Beath pin is drilled across the arm to pull the tendon/EndoButton construct into the tunnel (**Figure 5, C**).

For two-incision techniques, three small holes are made ulnar to the insertion hole for suture passage and tying (**Figure 5, D**). All bone debris is carefully irrigated to prevent heterotopic ossification.

Tendon Passage for Two Incisions

A curved Kelly clamp is used to carefully "hug" the radius from the anterior incision, directing the clamp toward the

FIGURE 3

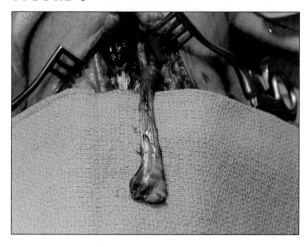

The ruptured distal biceps tendon has been retrieved from the wound and is being prepared for suture placement.

FIGURE 4

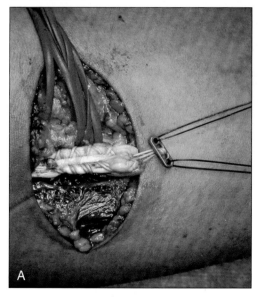
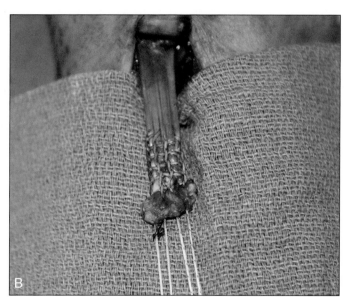

Tendon preparation. **A**, In the single-incision technique, an EndoButton is secured to the tendon. **B**, In the two-incision technique, different-colored No. 2 nonabsorbable sutures are passed in Krackow-type fashion to facilitate repair.

FIGURE 5

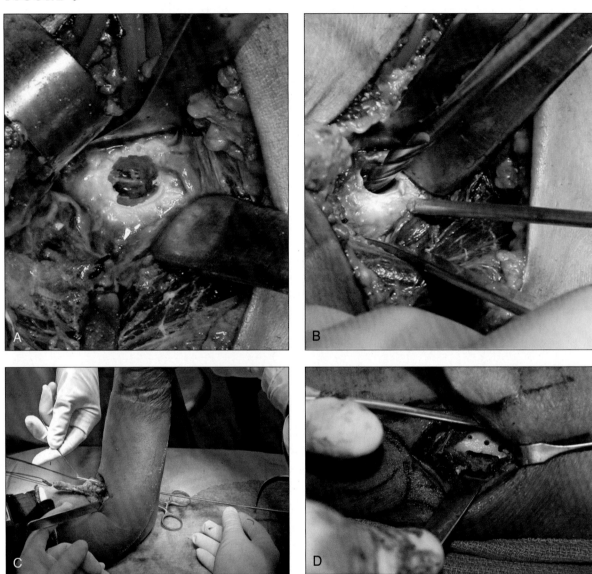

Radial tuberosity preparation. **A,** Intraoperative view from a single anterior incision in preparation for single-incision repair shows the drill hole made in the radial tuberosity. **B,** A 4.5-mm drill is used to penetrate the far cortex for the single-incision EndoButton repair. **C,** A Beath pin is drilled across the arm and used to pull the EndoButton sutures across the forearm and the tendon into the prepared hole. **D,** For the two-incision technique, a 1.5-cm trough is created to receive the tendon, and three small drill holes are made adjacent to the trough for suture passage. View is through the (dorsal) second incision.

dorsal forearm. The clamp is then used to push through the soft tissues and protrude the skin at the desired second incision site. The forearm is maintained in maximal pronation throughout this maneuver to keep the poste-

rior interosseous nerve as far away from potential injury as possible. The dorsal incision is then made overlying the Kelly clamp, carefully splitting through the extensor musculature and dissecting down to the radius (**Figure 6**).

Tendon Insertion and Securing

For single-incision techniques, the EndoButton is pulled through the radius and secured (**Figure 7, A**). Intraoperative fluoroscopy is used to confirm appropriate positioning of the EndoButton on the radial shaft (**Figure 7, B**). For the two-incision technique, the four suture ends from the tendon are then retrieved, carefully placed through the three small drill holes, and tied.

REHABILITATION

Postoperatively, the standard protocol consists of a hinged elbow brace with limited passive range of motion from full flexion to 30° of extension for the initial 2 weeks. The range is subsequently increased by 10° of extension every 2 weeks, until full extension is reached 6 weeks after surgery. Active-assisted and active range-of-motion exercises can begin at 8 weeks postoperatively (**Figure 8**). Cheung and associates[49] found that this rehabilitation protocol after a two-incision technique yielded excellent results, including mean Disabilities of the Arm, Shoulder and Hand (DASH) scores of 42.8 (range, 38 to 53), a mean loss of only 5.8° (range, 0° to 15°) of extension, no loss of flexion, a mean loss of only 3.5° (range, 0° to 10°) of pronation, and a mean loss of 8.1° (range, 0° to 15°) of supination. Flexion and supination strength were 91.4% (range, 83.3% to 100%) and 89.4% (range, 71.2% to 103%) of the uninjured side, respec-

FIGURE 6

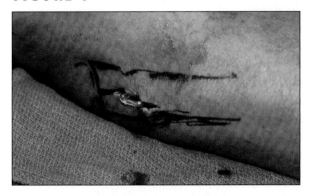

A Kelly clamp has been passed from the antecubital incision, carefully hugging the radius, and an incision over the dorsal forearm has been made.

FIGURE 7

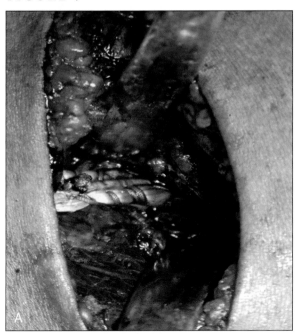
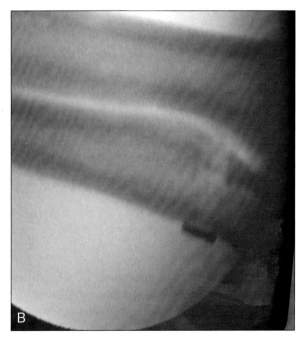

Tendon insertion and securing for single-incision technique. **A,** The repaired tendon is in the hole and appropriately tensioned. **B,** Intraoperative fluoroscopy confirms appropriate placement of the EndoButton.

FIGURE 8

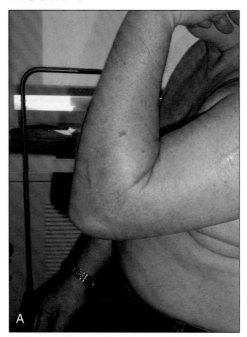 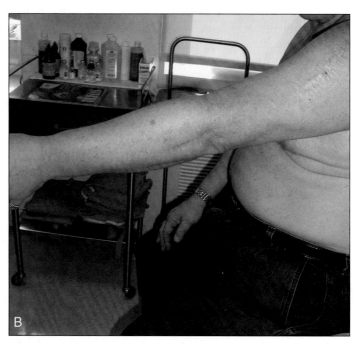

Flexion **(A)** and extension **(B)** at 8 weeks following a two-incision repair.

tively. The authors reported one case of rerupture in a patient who did not comply with the protocol. These reports are comparable to other published results of anatomic reinsertion of DBT ruptures.[3,11] Aggressive strengthening and higher-end plyometric activities should be avoided until 3 to 6 months, although running to maintain cardiovascular conditioning can begin in this time range. Return to contact sports and other upper extremity activity should be reserved until at least 6 months after surgery.[50]

CONCLUSIONS

Distal biceps ruptures are a relatively common injury and result from eccentric load on the biceps as typically seen when trying to lift a heavy object with one arm. They are more commonly seen in men and, if left detached, will lead to significant functional deficits—especially in supination and flexion. Both single- and double-incision techniques have been described to repair these injuries and both can lead to good functional outcomes; however, significant potential complications can occur with either technique.

REFERENCES

1. Giuffrè BM, Moss MJ: Optimal positioning for MRI of the distal biceps brachii tendon: Flexed abducted supinated view. *AJR Am J Roentgenol* 2004;182:944-946.
2. Lee HG: Traumatic avulsion of tendon of insertion of biceps brachii. *Am J Surg* 1951;82:290-292.
3. Morrey BF, Askew LJ, An KH, Dobyns JH: Rupture of the distal biceps tendon: Biomechanical assessment of different treatment options. *J Bone Joint Surg Am* 1985;67:418-421.
4. Seiler JG III, Parker LM, Chamberland PDC, Sherbourne GM, Carpenter WA: The distal biceps tendon: Two potential mechanisms involved in its rupture. Arterial supply and mechanical impingement. *J Shoulder Elbow Surg* 1995;4:149-156.
5. Safran MR, Graham SM: Distal biceps tendon ruptures: Incidence, demographics, and the effect of smoking. *Clin Orthop Relat Res* 2002;404:275-283.
6. Dobbie RP: Avulsion of the lower biceps brachii tendon: Analysis of 51 previously unreported cases. *Am J Surg* 1941;51:662-683.
7. Gilcreest EL: Rupture of muscle and tendons, particularly subcutaneous rupture of the biceps flexor cubiti. *JAMA* 1925;84:1819-1822.
8. Gilcreest EL: The common syndrome of rupture dislo-

cation and elongation at the long head of the biceps brachii: An analysis of 100 cases. *Surg Gynecol Obstet* 1934;58:322.

9. Rantanen J, Orava S: Rupture of the distal biceps tendon: A report of 19 patients treated with anatomic reinsertion and a meta-analysis of 147 cases found in the literature. *Am J Sports Med* 1999;27:128-132.

10. McKee MD, Hirji R, Schemitsch EH, Wild LM, Waddell JP: Patient-oriented functional outcome after repair of distal biceps tendon ruptures using a single incision technique. *J Shoulder Elbow Surg* 2005;14:302-306.

11. Bell RH, Wiley WB, Noble JS, Kuczynski DJ: Repair of distal biceps tendon ruptures. *J Shoulder Elbow Surg* 2000;9:223-226.

12. Ensslin S, Bauer GJ: Treatment of the avulsion of the distal biceps tendon by anatomic reinsertion with suture anchors by using limited anterior approach: A follow up of 24 patients. *Sportverletz Sportschaden* 2004;18:28-33.

13. Williams BD, Schweitzer ME, Weishaupt D, et al: Partial tears of the distal biceps tendon: MR appearance and associated clinical findings. *Skeletal Radiol* 2001;30:560-564.

14. Skaf AY, Boutin RD, Danta RW, et al: Bicipitoradial bursitis: MR imaging findings in 8 patients and anatomic data from contrast material opacification of bursae followed by routine radiographs and MR imaging in cadavers. *Radiology* 1999;212:111-116.

15. Meyer AW: Further evidences of attrition in the human body. *Am J Anat* 1924;34:24.

16. Strauch RJ, Michelson H, Rosenwasser MP: Repair of rupture of the distal biceps tendon of the biceps brachii. *Am J Orthop* 1997;26:151-156.

17. Ramsey ML: Distal biceps tendon injuries: Diagnosis and management. *J Am Acad Orthop Surg* 1999;7:199-207.

18. Morrey BF: Biceps tendon injury. *Instr Course Lect* 1999;48:405-410.

19. Ruland RT, Dunbar RP, Bowen JD: The biceps squeeze test for diagnosis of distal biceps tendon ruptures. *Clin Orthop Relat Res* 2005;437:128-131.

20. Falchook FS, Zlatkin MB, Erbacher GE, Moulton JS, Bisset GS, Murphy BJ: Rupture of the distal biceps tendon: Evaluation with MR imaging. *Radiology* 1994;190:659-663.

21. Vardakas DG, Musgrave DS, Varitimidis SE, Goebel F, Sotereanos DG: Partial rupture of the distal biceps tendon. *J Shoulder Elbow Surg* 2001;10:377-379.

22. Kelly EW, Steinmann S, O'Driscoll SW: Surgical treatment of partial distal biceps tendon ruptures through a single posterior incision. *J Shoulder Elbow Surg* 2003;12:456-461.

23. Dellaero DT, Mallon WJ: Surgical treatment of partial biceps tendon ruptures at the elbow. *J Shoulder Elbow Surg* 2006;15:215-217.

24. Bourne MH, Morrey BF: Partial rupture of the distal biceps tendon. *Clin Orthop Relat Res* 1991;271:143-148.

25. Davis WM, Yassine Z: An etiological factor in tear of the distal tendon of the biceps brachii: Report of two cases. *J Bone Joint Surg Am* 1956;39:1365-1368.

26. Hovelius L, Josefsson G: Rupture of the distal biceps tendon: Report of five cases. *Acta Orthop Scand* 1977;48:280-282.

27. Rokito AS, Mclaughlin MD, Gallagher MA, Zuckerman JD: Partial rupture of the distal biceps tendon. *J Shoulder Elbow Surg* 1996;5:73-75.

28. Durr HR, Stabler A, Pfahler M, Matzko M, Refior HJ: Partial rupture of the distal biceps tendon. *Clin Orthop Relat Res* 2000;374:195-200.

29. Ozturk K, Sahin V: Repair of distal biceps brachii tendon rupture: A case report. *Acta Orthop Traumatol Turc* 2002;36:167-171.

30. Kijowski R, Tuite M, Sanford M: Magnetic resonance imaging of the elbow: Part II. Abnormalities of the ligaments, tendons, and nerves. *Skeletal Radiol* 2005;34:1-18.

31. Chew ML, Giuffre BM: Disorders of the distal biceps brachii tendon. *Radiographics* 2005;25:1227-1237.

32. Miller TT, Adler RS: Sonography of tears of the distal biceps tendon. *AJR Am J Roentgenol* 2000;175:1081-1086.

33. Bell RH, Wiley WB, Noble JS, Kuczynski DJ: Repair of distal biceps brachii tendon ruptures. *J Shoulder Elbow Surg* 2000;9:223-226.

34. Sanchez-Sotelo J, Morrey BF, Adams RA, O'Driscoll SW: Reconstruction of chronic ruptures of the distal biceps tendon with use of an Achilles tendon allograft. *J Bone Joint Surg Am* 2002;84:999-1005.

35. Hallam P, Bain GI: Repair of chronic distal biceps tendon ruptures using autologous hamstring graft and the Endobutton. *J Shoulder Elbow Surg* 2004;13:648-651.

36. Levy HJ, Mashoof AA, Morgan D: Repair of chronic ruptures of the distal biceps tendon using flexor carpi radialis tendon graft. *Am J Sports Med* 2000;28:538-540.

37. Klonz A, Loitz D, Wohler P, Reilmann H: Rupture of the distal biceps tendon: Isokinetic power analysis and complications after anatomic reinsertion compared with fixation to the brachialis muscle. *J Shoulder Elbow Surg* 2003;12:607-611.

38. McReynolds IS: Avulsion of the insertion of the distal biceps brachii tendon and its surgical treatment. *J Bone Joint Surg Am* 1963;45:1780-1781.

39. Fischer WR, Shepanek LA: Avulsion of the insertion of the distal biceps brachii: Report of a case. *J Bone Joint Surg Am* 1956;38:158-159.

40. Meherin JM, Kilgore ES: The treatment of ruptures of the distal biceps brachii tendon. *Am J Surg* 1960;99:636-640.

41. Boyd HB, Anderson LD: A method for reinsertion of the distal biceps tendon. *J Bone Joint Surg Am* 1961;43:1041-1043.

42. Failla JM, Amadio PC, Morrey BF, et al: Proximal radioulnar synostosis after repair of distal biceps brachii rupture by the two-incision technique: Report of four cases. *Clin Orthop Relat Res* 1990;253:133-136.

43. Berlet GC, Johnson JA, Milne AD, Patterson SD, King GJ: Distal biceps tendon repair: An in vitro biomechanical study of tendon reattachment. *Am J Sports Med* 1998;26:428-432.

44. Barber FA, Herbert MA, Click JN: Suture anchor strength revisited. *Arthroscopy* 1996;12:32-38.

45. Wetzler MJ, Bartolozzi AR, Gillespie MJ, et al: Fatigue properties of suture anchors in anterior shoulder reconstructions: Mitek GII. *Arthroscopy* 1996;12:687-693.

46. Lemos SE, Ebramzedeh E, Kvitne RS: In vitro suture anchor fixation has superior yield strength to bone tunnel fixation for distal biceps tendon repair. *Am J Sports Med* 2004;32:406-410.

47. Sotereanos DG, Pierce TD, Varitimidis SE: A simplified method for repair of distal biceps tendon ruptures. *J Shoulder Elbow Surg* 2000;9:227-233.

48. El-Hawary R, MacDermid JC, Faber KJ, Patterson SD, King GJW: Distal biceps tendon repair: Comparison of surgical techniques. *J Hand Surg Am* 2003;28:496-502.

49. Cheung EV, Lazarus M, Taranta M: Immediate range of motion after distal biceps tendon repair. *J Shoulder Elbow Surg* 2005;14:516-518.

50. Curl LA: Return to sport following elbow surgery. *Clin Sports Med* 2004;23:353-366.

CHAPTER 4

TREATMENT OF TRICEPS INJURIES

BERNARD F. MORREY, MD

Ruptures of the triceps tendon are quite uncommon in athletes.[1-4] In fact, injuries to the triceps represented less than 1% of 856 upper extremity tendon injuries analyzed at the Mayo Clinic.[1] However, this injury is being increasingly recognized as a problem of total elbow arthroplasty,[2] and it has been associated with chronic disease states such as renal failure and associated hypoparathyroidism.[5] Most injuries occur as a result of trauma, either indirectly from a fall on the outstretched hand or, less commonly, from a direct blow. A recent survey of professional football players with triceps rupture covering a 7-year period identified 21 partial and complete injuries in 19 players.[6] The athletes at greatest risk are weight lifters. A relationship between triceps rupture and the use of anabolic steroids by athletes has been recognized.[7,8]

MECHANISM OF INJURY

Any one of the several variations of triceps insufficiency may occur after trauma or surgery, and some injuries can occur spontaneously. One uncommon mechanism of injury is a direct blow to the posterior aspect of the triceps at its insertion on the olecranon.[7,9,10] The most common location of the injury is at the attachment to the olecranon, but rarely the injury also occurs at the musculotendinous junction.[10]

Several conditions have been implicated to predispose disruption of the triceps attachment. These include such systemic disease processes as osteogenesis imperfecta tarda,[11] renal osteodystrophy, secondary hyperparathyroidism,[12,13] and chronic acidosis.[14] Tendon deficiencies have also been associated with steroid use for the man-

agement of lupus erythematosus[7] and in patients with diabetes and even Marfan syndrome.[17] The clinical setting currently most frequently associated with triceps insufficiency is total elbow arthroplasty.[2]

In spite of the association with debilitating states and conditions, triceps injury, although uncommon in this population, is well recognized to occur in the athletic population as well. Such diverse activities as power weightlifting and handball have been implicated.[7,8,18,19] The mechanism of injury is typically that of an eccentric contracture occurring in the process of resisting a force tending to flex the elbow. This often occurs with a fall on the outstretched hand. The classic example of this is the injury sustained in competitive weight lifters, usually during bench press. Poor conditioning and the use of anabolic steroids have also been implicated.[6,15] A less common mechanism resulting in the injury, not always localized to the tendinous attachment, is a direct blow.[17,20]

The frequency of occurrence has not been clearly defined. In a recent study of National Football League players, most of the individuals who sustained this injury were linemen, with the most common mechanism being eccentric loads to a contracting triceps mechanism, ie, a flexion force that overcomes the extension force generated by the triceps.[4] Interestingly, 7 patients actually had some symptoms before the acute event, and 5 of 19 had a history of a cortisone injection in the region before the documented rupture. Triceps injury can also occur in the skeletally immature athlete, most often as the result of an overuse syndrome.[21] Recognition of this fact has resulted in the development of rules that govern youth athletic performance. These typically prohibit

FIGURE 1

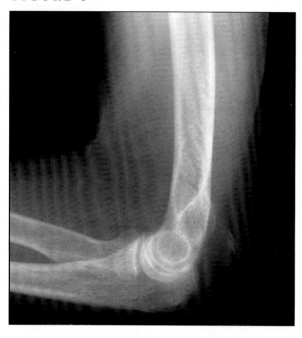

Lateral radiograph of the elbow of a patient with triceps rupture demonstrating an avulsed portion of olecranon. (Reproduced with permission from the Mayo Foundation, Rochester, MN.)

more than a 10% increase in the frequency of training over a 1-week period. In the adolescent, the elbow overuse injuries are most commonly seen in the throwing athlete.[21] As with other tendon pathology, however, acute rupture typically occurs in a tendon that has undergone degenerative changes. The injury can be associated with localized hematoma, and there are reports of ulnar nerve compression as a result of hematoma compression after triceps rupture in power weight lifters.[18,19]

EVALUATION

Without question, a history of acute pain and weakness in extension, and eccentric loading in flexion against forcible triceps contracture, represents the most reliable clinical feature assisting in making the diagnosis of triceps injury. Clinical examination reveals pain to palpation right at the site of the injury, which is usually at the insertion on the olecranon. Less commonly, pain is localized to the musculotendinous junction. It is not always possible to identify a palpable defect, but when present, this is a pathognomonic finding. If the injury occurs in

the musculotendinous junction, the symptoms are in the distal aspect of the brachium proximal to the elbow itself. Ecchymosis is not always present. Nonetheless, in all instances, some form of extension weakness is a reliable finding, although variable residual elbow extension strength function may be present. Typically, extension against gravity is not possible with a complete or extensive tear. Patients with partial tears are more likely to report pain with repetitive activity than single-event weakness.

The newer imaging modalities have assumed an increasingly important role in the diagnosis of triceps rupture, particularly partial rupture. In this setting, the pain does not markedly limit function, and delay before evaluation often occurs because some form of active function is possible.[19] The residual strength of extension is believed to be provided through the anconeus triceps mechanism. Individuals with complete rupture or extensive partial ruptures do have weakness that prevents extension of the arm against gravity.

Current imaging modalities can reliably make a definitive diagnosis that precisely defines the location and nature of the tear. Plain radiographs are extremely useful in those uncommon situations in which the triceps rupture is associated with an avulsed fleck of bone, which is readily identified on the lateral view[13,22] (**Figure 1**). The advent of MRI, however, has provided an accurate and reliable means of not only diagnosing this injury, but also localizing the site and the extent of the pathology[23,24] (**Figure 2**). Ultrasonography is also emerging as a reliable and less expensive imaging modality.[24]

PARTIAL RUPTURE

With triceps injury, the nature of the pathology is very much a function of the extent and duration of the injury. Several sites of failure have been documented, the least common of which is the musculotendinous junction.[25] The most common site by far is avulsion or detachment at the insertion of the olecranon.[6] More than 90% of these injuries do occur at the olecranon, with injury of the other sites being reported only occasionally.[11,26] At Mayo, we have found the tendinous central third is most typically detached with both complete and partial injury.[20] In individuals with chronic insufficiency, a delamination process has been observed that grossly and histologically resembles the pathology seen with a tear of the rotator cuff tendinous insertion.[27] In addition to the acute injury, other associated injuries may occasionally be present; concurrent fracture of the radial head has been described,[25,28] and one recent report of six such injuries indicates that the association of triceps ruptures with radial head fractures occurs more frequently than was previously appreciated.[29] Documentation of a fracture at the wrist along with triceps insufficiency indicates that both injuries can occur concurrently from a fall on the outstretched hand.[16]

TREATMENT

Treatment of triceps rupture may logically be categorized according to acute or chronic presentations and further stratified according to partial or complete ruptures. Partial tendon rupture frequently can be initially treated nonsurgically;[9] however, we have found in our experience at Mayo that a distinction must be made between a true partial rupture at the insertion and one occurring at the musculotendinous junction. A partial detachment from the olecranon does not heal reliably, if it ever heals. We do favor protecting the extremity and observing the amount of progress over a 6- to 8-week period. A strain of the attachment or of the musculotendinous junction will improve over this time period. Partial ruptures, while appearing to heal, will continue to be symptomatic with increased or high-demand activity, and unless clinical contraindications are present, surgical intervention is warranted. If, however, there is evidence of healing by progressive resolution of symptoms, then in our judgment this represents a strain, not a rupture, and nonsurgical management is recommended.

Surprisingly, the sensitivity of making the diagnosis during the acute stage is not markedly greater than during the chronic stage. In our experience dealing with a nonathletic population, a delayed repair offers virtually the same outcome as does a more acute intervention.[20] This observation may not be appropriately applied to a high-level athlete. Regardless, in our judgment immediate surgery is the treatment of choice for complete ruptures because these do not heal. At the time of exploration, the tendinous portion of the acute rupture is retracted.[28] Frequently, the interval between the ruptured tendon at its insertion develops a synovial bursal type of tissue that must be débrided. The retracted tendon must be mobilized and brought distally. Thus, delay in diagnosis and management results in a more difficult surgical procedure. However, complete disruption of the extensor mechanism is rela-

FIGURE 2

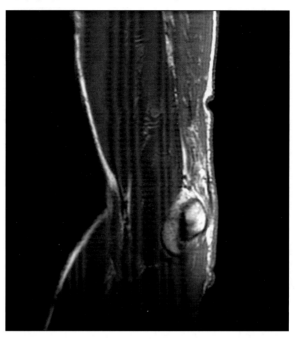

MRI revealing triceps rupture from its insertion. MRI is the most accurate imaging modality to make the diagnosis if the bone is not involved. (Reproduced with permission from the Mayo Foundation, Rochester, MN.)

tively uncommon; some form of continuity with the anconeus expansion is usually preserved. We use three techniques: direct reattachment (for acute injuries) and either anconeus rotation flap reconstruction or Achilles tendon allograft reconstruction in the delayed setting.[30]

Acute Repair

The treatment of choice for acute triceps tendon detachment is direct reattachment as soon as the diagnosis is made. We recommend avoiding delays of more than 2 or 3 weeks because of tendon retraction and resorption. Several techniques may be used to achieve the goal of direct reattachment.

Direct reattachment with nonabsorbable sutures though criss-crossed drill holes placed in the olecranon (**Figure 3**, *A*) is an effective treatment of acute ruptures. We use a heavy No. 5 nonabsorbable suture and place two parallel rows of running locked stitches in the tendinous portion of the triceps mechanism (**Figure 3**, *B* and *C*). The suture is then brought through cruciate drill

FIGURE 3

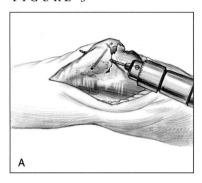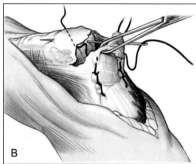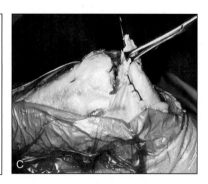

Direct reattachment technique for acute triceps tendon avulsion. **A,** Holes are placed in the proximal ulna in a criss-crossed and in a transverse pattern. **B,** For acute triceps tendon avulsion, No. 5 nonabsorbable running locked suture is passed through the avulsed tendon and into the olecranon through criss-crossed and transverse bone holes. **C,** The attachment of the anconeus to the lateral margin of the triceps allows the anconeus to serve as a reconstructive option for triceps deficiency. (Reproduced with permission from the Mayo Foundation, Rochester, MN.)

holes in the olecranon. With the elbow extended to 30°, the sutures are tied. To further ensure that the tendon is firmly approximated to its origin and to avoid poor healing from synovial fluid, a second transverse suture may be placed, which more securely applies the tendon to its site of attachment. If there has been any delay in the treatment, the adventitial bursa tissue should be removed and the area scarified to ensure healing.

Delayed Reconstruction

If the acute injury is not recognized initially, then some form of reconstruction is required. In our practice, we use two techniques. One involves rotation of the anconeus from the ulna and from the humerus. The fascial expansion of the anconeus at the triceps allows continuity of the extensor mechanism to be centered over the olecranon. This enhances the alignment and mechanical advantage of the triceps mechanism. The remaining torn portions of the tendon are secured to the tendon remnants. The second technique is reconstruction using Achilles tendon allograft, which is described below. Bennett and others[31,32] have described a forearm fascial flap to reconstruct the triceps mechanism, and the classic triceps fascial turndown procedure is well known to many, but these are not as reliable in our opinion.

Anconeus Rotation Technique
With the patient supine, the arm is brought across the chest. The interval between the anconeus and the exten-

sor carpi ulnaris is identified. The anconeus is mobilized from its bed on the lateral margin of the proximal ulna and from its humeral origin in continuity with the triceps (**Figure 4,** *A*). The complex is elevated from the capsule and the triceps/anconeal sleeve is mobilized from lateral to medial to cover the olecranon process (**Figure 4,** *B* and *C*). The sleeve of extensor musculature is secured in the manner described above, with criss-crossed No. 5 nonabsorbable suture (**Figure 4,** *D*). The suture is tied with the elbow at 30° of extension.

One important step is to recognize that the anconeus is left attached distally and mobilized sufficiently medial to fully cover the site of triceps attachment. The tendinous fibers that are displaced medially are rotated under the tendon and sewn to themselves.

Achilles Tendon Allograft
It is uncommon that an Achilles tendon allograft is required in the athletic population, as this technique is most commonly of value in grossly neglected ruptures or in those in whom the deficiency has resulted from surgical débridement, such as is seen with the management of a septic joint. In settings of marked tissue loss or retraction of the triceps, an Achilles tendon allograft is an effective means of bridging the gap (**Figure 5,** *A* and *B*). This reconstruction is effective as a salvage type of operation but would not be considered reliable in allowing a competitive athlete to return to sport.

The patient is placed supine and the arm is brought across the chest. The incision begins approximately 4 cm

FIGURE 4

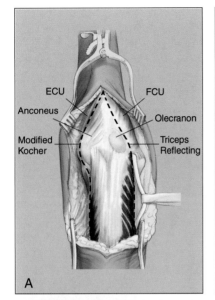

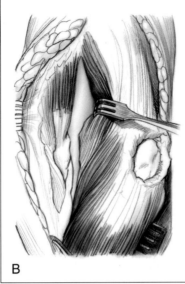

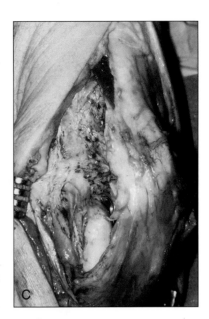

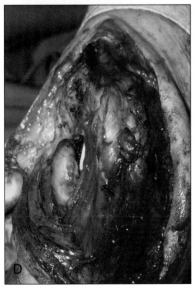

Anconeus rotation technique. **A,** The anconeus origin from the lateral margin of the triceps is shown. **B,** If the deficit in the triceps tendon is not too extensive, the anconeus may be mobilized and oriented over the tip of the olecranon. **C** and **D,** The tear or deficiency is repaired or reinforced with No. 5 nonabsorbable suture. ECU = extensor carpi ulnaris, FCU = flexor carpi ulnaris. (Reproduced with permission from the Mayo Foundation, Rochester, MN.)

distal to the olecranon and extends proximally to the extent necessary to identify the distal third of the triceps musculature. The ulnar nerve is identified and protected. The defect is débrided, and the triceps musculature is mobilized and its flexibility is tested.

There are two modes of attachment of the Achilles tendon allograft to the proximal ulna. One involves a chevron resection of the proximal olecranon. A matching preparation of the calcaneal bone allows an

osseous union of the distal site. The calcaneus is fashioned in a way to match the preparation of the proximal ulna (**Figure 5,** *C*). The calcaneus is secured as an allograft to the olecranon with a cancellous screw (**Figure 5,** *D* and *E*). The alternative attachment consists of preparing a trough in the subcutaneous border of the proximal ulna. The calcaneal component of the Achilles graft is removed, and the tubular portion of the Achilles tendon allograft is inserted in the trough

FIGURE 5

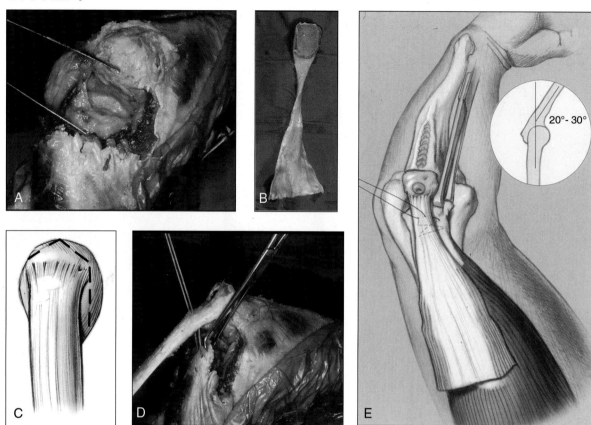

A, An Achilles tendon allograft provides an ideal reconstructive unit, especially if the defect is significant. If the olecranon is also deficient the calcaneus attachment is used **(B)** and is fashioned and secured to the olecranon with a screw **(C, and D)** or the allograft tendon is placed in a trough created in the subcutaneous border of the ulna. **E,** With the elbow at 20° to 30° flexion, the triceps is brought distally and the Achilles fascia is brought proximally and secured. The proximal aspect of the graft is secured with multiple No. 1 interrupted and running sutures. (Reproduced with permission from the Mayo Foundation, Rochester, MN.)

and then secured with nonabsorbable sutures placed through bone holes.

In the athlete, the olecranon is typically intact, so the calcaneal portion of the allograft is not necessary. A trough is made in the subcutaneous border of the proximal ulna and the tendinous portion of the Achilles graft is inserted into the tendinous trough. Two drill holes are placed through the proximal ulna and through the tendon, thus securing it to its bed of insertion. The elbow is placed in 30° of extension. The triceps musculature is mobilized as far distally as possible. The fascia is brought as far proximal as possible under tension and a No. 5 nonabsorbable suture is used to secure the midportion of the triceps, often with a portion of its residual tendon, to the

midportion of the graft at the site identified by the proximal and distal retraction of the two tissues. Once the No. 5 nonabsorbable suture has been placed and secured, the elbow is brought into full extension, relaxing the graft. The triceps tendon is brought distally and the tendon is secured to the muscle and fascia of the triceps with running absorbable suture. Closure is routine.

Revision

An uncommon but real clinical issue is the management of the failed repair. In our experience, if the initial repair is unsuccessful, the site of attachment will undergo degenerative or inflammatory changes. We have been successful in revisions by using heavy No. 5 nonabsorbable suture

FIGURE 6

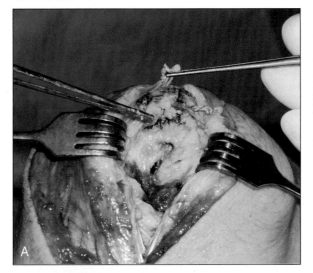

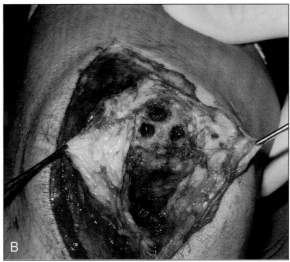

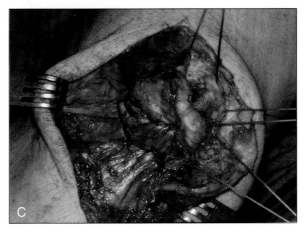

Revision for failed triceps tendon repair in a professional football player. **A,** Failed reattachment resulted in a marked synovitis. **B,** The triceps was débrided and the bed prepared. **C,** The triceps tendon was then mobilized and successfully reattached through drill holes in the olecranon. (Reproduced with permission from the Mayo Foundation, Rochester, MN.)

placed through bone holes. The preparation of the osseous bed is important, as is the débridement of the degenerative and bursal-type tissue (**Figure 6**).

REHABILITATION

In all instances, the elbow is placed in an anterior splint in approximately 30° of extension. This position is maintained for approximately 3 weeks. Following this, active flexion to 90° is allowed, with extension being active-assisted, principally using gravity. Full flexion is allowed over the next 3 weeks and is fully realized within 6 weeks of surgery. If there is confidence in the repair/reconstruction, active extension with the assistance of gravity is allowed at this time. After 6 weeks, if healing appears to

have progressed, the patient may gradually begin extending the elbow against gravity. This is done without weights other than that of the forearm. After an additional 2 weeks, if progress has been maintained, gentle extension weights are allowed beginning at 1 lb (2.2 kg). In a graduated program of extension, weightlifting is allowed from 3 to 6 months, with aggressive progression to normal activity from 6 to 12 months. Typically, approximately 80% of normal strength would be anticipated at approximately 3 months in the acute setting. At 6 months, approximately 90% of the strength will have returned. We do, however, advise patients that it takes a full year for a complete recovery after triceps injury. It is possible that the healing period would be abbreviated, but in many instances it is more prolonged than would ordinarily be expected.

OUTCOMES

In general, the management of either delayed or acute repair of triceps deficiency has been quite effective in restoring function.[12,30] In most instances, improvement of strength allows extension against gravity and normal motion is restored. A minimal loss of 5° to 10° of terminal extension may be observed, however. In our experience, surprisingly good results have been observed with either the repair or reconstruction even after delays of up to a year.[30] As mentioned above, the patient should be informed that the recovery may be slow. Unlike distal biceps tendon injury, the recovery period from triceps repair may take at least a year to be fully realized. Typically, protected function is recommended for the first 3 months.

Van Riet and associates[20] and Celli and associates[2] conducted a comprehensive assessment of Mayo's 20-year experience with 37 triceps deficiencies, which included 23 triceps injuries and 14 repairs and reconstructions that occurred after elbow arthroplasty.[2] Of the 23 not related to joint arthroplasty, 8 were partial and 15 were complete ruptures. Only two (8%) had osseous avulsions. Of these 23, 14 were primary repairs and 9 were reconstructions, and these were followed for an average of 88 months. At final follow-up, the average arc of motion was 10° to 135°. Two patients lacked a functional arc of motion, but both had degenerative arthrosis of the elbow. Isokinetic and dynamic testing in 10 patients showed that the peak strength was approximately 82% of the uninvolved extremity. The endurance, however, was almost 99% of normal. Of particular interest, results from repair and reconstruction were comparable but the recovery period was prolonged in those undergoing reconstruction. Overall, 90% were considered to have had a subjective satisfactory outcome and all patients were able to extend against gravity.

AUTHOR'S PREFERENCE

The approach used at Mayo has been outlined above. In the acute tear, we repair sooner rather than later. A posterior incision just lateral to the midline is performed. The ulnar nerve is identified but is not decompressed. A No. 5 nonabsorbable suture in a running locked stitch is placed down the medial and lateral aspects of the central portion of the tendon, which is the part that is most commonly torn. With the elbow in 30° of extension, the triceps is repaired to the freshened site of detachment using two criss-crossed drill holes placed in the proximal ulna. A second transverse suture is then placed across the olecranon and a locked stitch is inserted in the tendon just at the tendinous attachment site to the ulna. If a fracture has occurred and the tendon is avulsed, depending upon its size, this may be fixed using two Kirschner wires enhanced with figure-of-8 tension band wiring. If the injury is chronic and the deficiency can no longer be immobilized and reliably attached directly, then we favor the anconeus rotation technique described above. The Achilles tendon allograft technique is resorted to only when the anconeus is not present or when the deficiency is so great as to require tissue augmentation.

REFERENCES

1. Anzel SH, Covey KW, Weiner AD, Lipscomb PR: Disruption of muscles and tendons: An analysis of 1,014 cases. *Surgery* 1959;45:406-414.
2. Celli A, Arash A, Adams RA, Morrey BF: Triceps insufficiency following total elbow arthroplasty. *J Bone Joint Surg Am* 2005;87:1957-1964.
3. Gilcreest EL: Rupture of muscles and tendons. *JAMA* 1925;84:1819.
4. O'Reilly KP, Warhol MJ, Meredith CN, et al: Immediate and delayed ultrastructural changes in skeletal muscle following eccentric exercise. *Med Sci Sports Exerc* 1986;18(Suppl):S42.
5. Tsourvakas S, Gouvalas K, Gimtsas C, Tsianas N, Founta P, Ameridis N: Bilateral and simultaneous rupture of the triceps tendon in chronic renal failure and secondary hyperparathyroidism. *Arch Orthop Trauma Surg* 2004;124:278-280.
6. Mair SD, Isbell WM, Gill TJ, Schlegel TF, Hawkins RJ: Triceps tendon ruptures in professional football players. *Am J Sports Med* 2004;32:431-434.
7. Sherman OH, Snyder SJ, Fox JM: Triceps tendon avulsion in a professional body builder: A case report. *Am J Sports Med* 1984;12:328-329.
8. Louis DS, Peck D: Triceps avulsion fracture in a weightlifter. *Orthopedics* 1992;15:207-211.
9. Anderson KJ, LeCocq JF: Rupture of the triceps tendon. *J Bone Joint Surg Am* 1957;39:444-446.
10. O'Driscoll SW: Intramuscular triceps rupture. *Can J Surg* 1992;35:203-206.
11. Match RM, Corrylos EV: Bilateral avulsion fracture of the triceps tendon insertion from skiing with osteogenesis imperfecta tarda. *Am J Sports Med* 1983;11:99-102.
12. Cirincione RJ, Baker BE: Tendon ruptures with secondary hyperparathyroidism: A case report. *J Bone Joint Surg Am* 1975;57:852-853.

13. Fery A, Sommelet J, Schmitt D, Lipp B: Avulsion bilaterale simultanee des tendons quadricipital et rotulien et rupture du tendon tricipital chez un hemodialyse hyperparathyroidien. *Rev Chir Orthop Reparatrice Appar Mot* 1978;64:175-181.

14. Murphy KJ, McPhee I: Tears of major tendons in chronic acidosis with elastosis. *J Bone Joint Surg Am* 1965;47:1253-1258.

15. Maydl K: Ueber subcutane Muskel- und Sehnenzerreissungen, sowie Rissfracturen, mit Berücksichtigung der analogen, durch directe Gewalt enstandenen und offenen Verletzungen. *Dtsch Z Chir* 1882;17:306.

16. Levy M, Fishel RE, Stern GM: Triceps tendon avulsion with or without fracture of the radial head: A rare injury? *J Trauma* 1978;18:677-679.

17. Penhallow DP: Report of a case of ruptured triceps due to direct violence. *NY Med J* 1910;91:76.

18. Duchow J, Kelm J, Kohn D: Acute ulnar nerve compression syndrome in a powerlifter with triceps tendon rupture: A case report. *Int J Sports Med* 2000;21:308-310.

19. Herrick RT, Herrick S: Ruptured triceps in a powerlifter presenting as cubital tunnel syndrome: A case report. *Am J Sports Med* 1987;15:514-516.

20. van Riet RP, Morrey BF, Ho E, O'Driscoll SWL: Surgical treatment of distal triceps ruptures. *J Bone Joint Surg Am* 2003;85:1961-1967.

21. Gill TJ IV, Micheli LJ: The immature athlete: Common injuries and overuse syndromes of the elbow and wrist. *Clin Sports Med* 1996;15:401-423.

22. Preston FS, Adicoff A: Hyperparathyroidism with avulsion at three major tendons. *N Engl J Med* 1962;266:968-971.

23. Fritz RC, Steinbach LS: Magnetic resonance imaging of the musculoskeletal system: Part 3. The elbow. *Clin Orthop Relat Res* 1996;324:321-339.

24. Popovic N, Ferrara MA, Daenen B, Georis P, Lemaire R: Imaging overuse injury of the elbow in professional team handball players: A bilateral comparison using plain films, stress radiography, ultrasound, and magnetic resonance imaging. *Int J Sports Med* 2001;22:60-67.

25. Morrey BF: Rupture of the triceps tendon, in Morrey BF (ed): *The Elbow and Its Disorders*, ed 3. Philadelphia, PA, WB Saunders Co, 2000.

26. Gerard F, Marion A, Garbuio P, Tropet Y: Distal traumatic avulsion of the triceps brachii: Apropos of a treated case. *Chir Main* 1998;17:321-324.

27. Searfoss R, Tripi J, Bowers W: Triceps brachii rupture: Case report. *J Trauma* 1976;16:244-246.

28. Pantazopoulos T, Exarchou E, Stavrou Z, Hartofilakidis-Garofalidis G: Avulsion of the triceps tendon. *J Trauma* 1975;15:827-829.

29. Inhofe PD, Moneim MS: Late presentation of triceps rupture: A case report and review of the literature. *Am J Orthop* 1996;25:790-792.

30. Sanchez-Sotelo J, Morrey BF: Surgical techniques for reconstruction of chronic insufficiency of the triceps: Rotation flap using anconeus and tendo Achilles allograft. *J Bone Joint Surg Br* 2002;84:1116-1120.

31. Bennett BS: Triceps tendon rupture: Case report and a method of repair. *J Bone Joint Surg Am* 1961;44:741-744.

32. Clayton ML, Thirupathi RG: Rupture of the triceps tendon with olecranon bursitis: A case report with a new method of repair. *Clin Orthop Relat Res* 1984;184:183-185.

CHAPTER 5

MEDIAL COLLATERAL LIGAMENT RECONSTRUCTION

GUILLEM GONZALEZ-LOMAS, MD
NEAL ELATTRACHE, MD
CHRISTOPHER S. AHMAD, MD

High-level athletes generate tremendous valgus stresses at the elbow during the late cocking and acceleration phases of throwing. Indeed, biomechanical studies have estimated that valgus moments during those phases attain 120 N·m.[1] The primary restraint to valgus forces at the elbow is the anterior bundle of the medial collateral ligament (MCL). As such, the large tensile forces it endures place it at risk for injury. Waris[2] first recognized and described MCL injuries in javelin throwers in 1946. The injury often presaged the end of a throwing career. In 1974, Jobe and associates[3] developed a technique for MCL reconstruction that altered this bleak outlook. The technique involved transection and reflection of the flexor-pronator mass, transposing the ulnar nerve submuscularly, and reconstructing the MCL with a tendon graft through bone holes that traversed two cortices of both the humerus and ulna. Since its inception, the technique has proven successful in restoring elite throwers to preinjury levels of performance. The procedure is, however, technically demanding and fraught with several potential complications. More recent techniques have attempted to address these shortcomings. Moreover, newer biomechanical studies have furthered our understanding of the dynamic properties of the MCL.[4] This chapter reviews the pathophysiology of MCL injuries, analyzes the available reconstruction techniques, and summarizes relevant outcome studies.

FUNCTIONAL ANATOMY AND BIOMECHANICS

Elbow stability results from a static and dynamic interplay of bony anatomy, ligamentous restraints, and surrounding musculature. Interlocking of the bony anatomy governs stability in <20° of extension and >120° of flexion (olecranon in olecranon fossa).[5] In the arc of 20° to 120°, which is the functional arc of throwing, however, ligamentous restraints provide the majority of elbow stability.[4] The MCL complex represents the ligamentous restraint to valgus force at the elbow. It is composed of three ligaments—the anterior oblique ligament (AOL), the posterior oblique ligament, and the transverse ligament. The AOL is the strongest of these and withstands the bulk of valgus force. It originates on the humerus, distal to the axis of rotation, and inserts on the ulnar side of the coronoid process near the sublime tubercle. The AOL can be further subdivided anatomically. Its anterior and posterior bands provide a reciprocal function in resisting valgus stress through the range of flexion-extension motion (ie, the anterior band is taut in extension, the posterior band in flexion.).[6] It also divides itself into intracapsular and extracapsular components. One AOL component lies within the medial capsule. The other lies on the superficial surface of the capsule that, in addition, serves as a partial origin for the flexor digitorum superficialis (FDS).

During overhead throwing sports like baseball, water polo, javelin throwing, and tennis, enormous valgus forces are generated across the elbow. The calculated valgus stress across the elbow in elite athletes has been calculated as 64 N·m in baseball pitchers[7,8] and 60 N·m during a tennis serve.[9,10] The static demand on the MCL in resisting valgus torque during baseball pitching has been reported at 35 N·m.[7] These forces exceed the known tensile strength of cadaveric MCL specimens, which is

33 N·m.[8] Accordingly, the MCL is at risk for injury during repetitive throwing. The excess valgus stress is likely dissipated among a combination of the surrounding muscular, ligamentous, and osseous structures. Surrounding musculature, for example, plays a critical role in elbow stability during valgus stress. Park and Ahmad[11] demonstrated in a cadaveric model that the flexor carpi ulnaris is a primary dynamic contributor to valgus stability and the FDS is a secondary stabilizer, in addition to sharing an origin with the MCL. Because there is a significant muscular contribution to elbow stability, muscle morbidity must be minimized during surgical reconstruction.

Although soft-tissue structures act primarily as stabilizers during the functional arc of throwing, the bony anatomy of the elbow still plays an important stabilizing role during this range of motion. In particular, biomechanical evidence strongly suggests that the interlocking of the olecranon in the olecranon fossa contributes to elbow stability. The phenomenon of posteromedial olecranon impingement arises as a result of valgus stress during throwing, which drives the posteromedial edge of the olecranon into the olecranon fossa. Andrews and Timmerman[12] reported that elbow valgus instability developed in 25% of professional baseball players after olecranon débridement for posteromedial impingement. Kamineni and associates[13] examined the effect of resection of the posteromedial olecranon on elbow instability biomechanically. They demonstrated that stepwise resection of the olecranon leads to a stepwise increase in elbow valgus angulation. Another study concluded that strain on the AOL increased with olecranon resection greater than 3 mm.[14] The suggestion was that aggressive olecranon débridement could lead to MCL instability. Ahmad and associates[15] demonstrated that the converse could also occur; ie, subtle instability can lead to posteromedial olecranon impingement and eventually osteophyte formation. Other studies have provided compelling evidence that loss of valgus stability can lead to additional pathology such as ulnar neuritis, radiocapitellar arthrosis, and loose bodies.[16]

HISTORY

The primary symptom in patients with MCL injuries is pain during the acceleration phase of throwing. In addition, patients may report loss of velocity, accuracy, and stamina while throwing. A complete history should document previous elbow problems, injections, and surgery. The examiner must differentiate acute injuries from chronic symptoms. Athletes with acute MCL tears will report a sudden onset of pain with or without a "popping" sensation that occurred during a particular throw. Often, they will report being unable to continue throwing. With acute MCL injuries, the resulting hemorrhage and injury can compress the neighboring ulnar nerve. As a result, symptoms of ulnar nerve irritation, including pain and numbness in the ipsilateral ring and little fingers, may present concurrently.

Complete disruption of the MCL can also lead to chronic valgus instability. In contradistinction to those with acute injuries, athletes with chronic MCL injuries report insidious pain and soreness along the inner elbow during throwing rather than recalling a specific traumatic event. Often these patients report bouts of soreness that arise during and after throwing that respond to nonsurgical management. Ultimately, most present when they can no longer throw at 75% of their baseline speed. Athletes will describe this as a loss of "zip" or "pop" in their throwing.

Occasionally a chronic injury underlies a superimposed acute injury. In these instances, the athlete will recount a chronic MCL history punctuated by a sudden, isolated giving way or medial elbow pain that prompted a visit to the clinic.

PHYSICAL EXAMINATION

The physical examination must include inspection, palpation, and examination of bilateral upper extremity range of motion and stability. Pathology in the shoulder and scapula may uncover hidden improper throwing mechanics. Examination for the presence of the palmaris is needed if an MCL reconstruction is planned. Positive findings for MCL injury include point tenderness to palpation 2 cm distal to the medial epicondyle (reported in up to 80% of athletes undergoing reconstruction)[17] and painful valgus instability, as well as positive MCL-specific tests.

Several tests are available to examine the integrity of the MCL. The classic test is to stress the elbow at 30° of flexion while stabilizing the humerus, because this removes the bony interlocking effect of elbow stability. This test is positive when the patient reports pain and the medial joint space opens up in response to valgus stress. The "milking maneuver" involves having the ath-

FIGURE 1

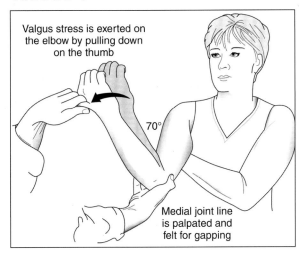

Modified milking maneuver. (Adapted with permission from Safran MR: Injury to the UCL: Diagnosis and treatment. *Sports Med Arthrosc Rev* 2003;11:15-24.)

FIGURE 2

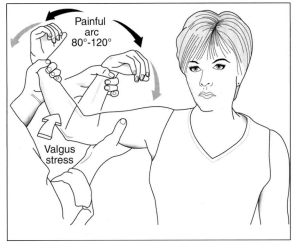

Moving valgus stress test for MCL injury, recently described by O'Driscoll and associates.[20] The patient's elbow is brought into abduction and external rotation. The examiner flexes and extends the patient's elbow while applying a valgus force at the elbow. In the patient with an MCL injury, this should reproducibly cause pain in the arc between 80° and 120°. (Adapted with permission from Safran MR: Injury to the UCL: Diagnosis and treatment. *Sports Med Arthrosc Rev* 2003;11:15-24.)

lete valgus stress his or her own elbow. The athlete flexes the affected elbow beyond 90°, with the hand in a "thumbs up" position, and brings the contralateral hand under the arm of the affected elbow to grab the extended thumb.[18] While the athlete pulls on his or her own thumb, stressing the medial elbow, the examiner palpates the MCL for tenderness, joint space opening, and end point. The affected elbow is compared with the normal, contralateral side. Relative differences in laxity must be interpreted with caution because elite throwers may demonstrate relatively more laxity in the throwing elbow than in the contralateral elbow at asymptomatic baseline.[19] Therefore, the examination should be more focused on eliciting pain and lack of an end point. In a modification of the milking maneuver illustrated in **Figure 1**, the surgeon performs the valgus stress by pulling on the patient's thumb with one hand while holding the elbow with the other hand.[16] One shortcoming of the milking maneuver is that the patient will often flex the affected elbow >120°. At this degree of flexion, the bony anatomy begins to contribute to elbow stability. To address this, O'Driscoll and associates[20] recently described another test, the moving valgus stress test. In this test, the examiner places the athlete's shoulder in abduction and external rotation. The examiner holds the athlete's forearm with one hand and the humerus with the other while flexing and extending the elbow

and applying a valgus stress, as shown in **Figure 2**. If the MCL is injured, the athlete will experience pain in the arc of 80° to 120°. One advantage of this technique is that the examiner can also control external rotation of the shoulder, which has classically been a confounding factor in tests of elbow stability. Additionally, the test more accurately mimics the position of the elbow during throwing. Two points should be emphasized concerning this maneuver: First, cadaveric studies have verified that the best position to demonstrate valgus laxity is with the forearm in neutral rotation during testing;[21] and second, the expected amount of laxity in an elbow with complete MCL disruption will be subtle, at most a few millimeters.

Care must be taken to rule out associated injuries, in particular flexor-pronator mass avulsions. Several authors have reported significant coexistence of flexor-pronator ruptures with acute MCL tears.[22,23] Athletes with these combined injuries will have tenderness at the medial epicondyle origin that worsens with resisted wrist flexion. The ulnar nerve should also be examined for concurrent neuritis by attempting to elicit a Tinel sign.

FIGURE 3

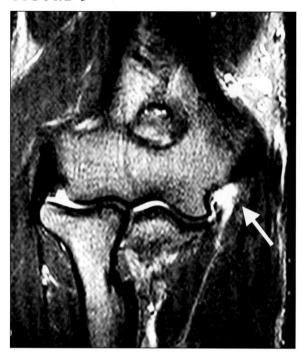

T2-weighted MRI scan of elbow. Arrow indicates MCL tear.

IMAGING STUDIES

Imaging modalities can help in delineating the diagnosis of MCL tears. AP, lateral, and axillary radiographs without valgus stress can be obtained to rule out the presence of osteochondral lesions, loose bodies, and osteophytes. Stress radiographs can assess instability in the case of an acute MCL tear. Significant radiographic elbow valgus laxity can exist in the dominant, asymptomatic throwing arm of pitchers: up to 0.5 mm of laxity has been measured in professional baseball pitchers.[19] Commercially available stress devices are available that boast a reported 94% sensitivity and 100% specificity for MCL tears.[24] Nevertheless, even in the normal, nonthrowing population, the difference in elbow valgus laxity between normal elbows can be up to 0.5 mm. Therefore, diagnosing MCL injury based on laxity may not be reliable. Although some authors have found that ~2 mm of increased relative valgus laxity denotes an MCL tear,[17,25] others have reported that <50% of athletes who underwent warranted MCL reconstruction had positive stress radiographs.[26]

MRI may help define the extent of MCL injury (**Figure 3**). It visualizes the ligament directly and can help identify coexisting pathology such as in the radiocapitellar joint. MRI sensitivity has been reported to be between 57% and 79%, whereas specificity has been found to range from 79% to 100%.[26,27] MR arthrography has more reliable sensitivity (92%) and specificity (100%).[28] MRI using a high-field closed magnet, thin-slice images, and enhanced with intra-articular gadolinium contrast appears to have dependable diagnostic value.

Dynamic ultrasonography has also been studied as a diagnostic tool for MCL tears.[29,30] Although this modality is noninvasive and inexpensive, accurate diagnosis is operator-dependent.

INDICATIONS/ CONTRAINDICATIONS

In deciding whether to operate on an athlete, the surgeon must consider the athlete's individual demands, goals, and expectations along with the degree of MCL injury. Initial nonsurgical treatment should consist of 6 weeks of complete rest from throwing while undergoing a flexor-pronator strengthening program. If after 6 weeks the patient is asymptomatic and has a normal examination, then a gradual return to throwing is begun. At this point, patients can also benefit from a structured throwing mechanics optimization program. Rettig and associates[31] demonstrated a 42% return to preinjury level of play with nonsurgical management lasting an average of 24.5 weeks.

The primary indication for surgical MCL reconstruction is a diagnosis of MCL insufficiency that has failed nonsurgical treatment. The diagnosis of MCL insufficiency is arrived at from a thorough history, physical examination, and interpretation of imaging as outlined above. Patients who meet these criteria and who would like to undergo reconstruction must be informed of and prepared to undergo extensive and lengthy postoperative rehabilitation.

Patients contraindicated for surgical MCL reconstruction include those with asymptomatic tears and those who do not wish to continue throwing at a high level or who cannot participate in the significant postoperative rehabilitation required. Patients with coexisting ulnohumeral or radiocapitellar arthritis should be informed of the possibility of continued or worsening pain following reconstruction.

RECONSTRUCTION TECHNIQUES

Modified Jobe Technique

This technique is usually done using a sterile tourniquet on the upper arm. A 10-cm incision centered over the medial epicondyle is made. Care is taken to protect the sensory branches of the medial antebrachial cutaneous nerve, just anterior to the medial epicondyle. The flexor-pronator mass is then divided longitudinally along its fibers by incising the raphe from the medial epicondyle to the sublime tubercle (**Figure 4,** *A*). The flexor-pronator muscle mass is separated from the MCL with an elevator. At this point, the ligament can be inspected and examined by stressing the elbow in valgus at 30° of elbow flexion. The ligament is split longitudinally to visualize the ulnohumeral joint (**Figure 4,** *B* and *C*). If the MCL is insufficient, the ulnohumeral articulation will open. Converging 3.2-mm drill holes are made in the ulna anterior and posterior to the sublime tubercle, leaving at least 5 mm of bone bridge between the holes (**Figure 4,** *D* and *E*). The drill holes are connected with an angled curette.

A 4.5-mm drill hole is made on the medial epicondyle, at the site of the anatomic origin of the anterior bundle of the MCL. The hole is made in the anterior cortex and does not penetrate the posterior cortex of the humerus (**Figure 4,** *F*). The fascia over the anterior aspect of the epicondyle is split superior to the last hole to expose the broad, flat surface of the anterosuperior epicondyle. Two 3.2-mm drill holes are then made. The first is drilled just anterior to the epicondylar attachment of the medial intermuscular septum (superior and anterior to the 4.5-mm hole) and directed to communicate with the 4.5-mm drill hole in the medial epicondyle. The second 3.2-mm drill hole is made in the anterosuperior surface of the epicondyle, approximately 1 cm posterior to the previous 3.2-mm hole.

The palmaris longus from the ipsilateral arm is harvested through a series of small transverse incisions beginning at the distal flexor crease of the wrist. Additional skin incisions are made 7.5 and 15 cm from the wrist, exposing the entire length of the tendon. Alternatively, the palmaris longus may be harvested with a tendon stripper and a single incision in the flexor crease of the wrist. A No. 2 nonabsorbable suture is cross-stitched at each end of the graft. The graft is passed through the proximal ulnar bone tunnel and medial epicondyle in a figure-of-8 configuration. With the elbow placed in varus stress and 60° of flexion, and the forearm in supination, tension is applied to the graft. The ulnar side of the graft is sutured to the remnants of the MCL adjacent to the sublime tubercle. The proximal limb of the graft is sutured to the medial intermuscular septum outside the drill hole on the superior surface of the epicondyle. Simple sutures are placed in the crossing limbs of the graft, further tensioning the graft and enhancing fixation. The native ligament is then repaired over the graft with simple sutures placed. **Figure 4,** *G* illustrates the final construct. The muscle fascia is repaired, and the skin is closed.

Docking Technique

The docking technique modifies the Jobe technique further, simplifying graft passage, tensioning, and fixation (**Figure 5,** *A*). The initial approach to the ulna closely parallels the Jobe technique. The flexor-pronator mass is split and elevated from the MCL and the ulnar tunnel is made in the fashion described above. The humeral tunnel position is located in the anterior half of the medial epicondyle at the anatomic insertion of the native MCL, similar to the Jobe technique. This tunnel is created to a depth of 15 mm using a 4-mm burr or drill. The upper border of the epicondyle is exposed by excising the fascia there. Two small exit tunnels separated by a bone bridge of 5 mm to 1 cm are created, stemming from the 4-mm primary humeral tunnel. Suture loops are then placed with a straight needle from the primary humeral tunnel through the exit tunnels to facilitate graft passage (**Figure 5,** *B*). With the elbow in forearm supination and mild varus stress, the horizontal incision in the native MCL is repaired with a No. 2.0 absorbable suture.

The graft is then passed through the ulnar tunnel from anterior to posterior (**Figure 5,** *C*). The posterior limb of the graft is passed into the humeral tunnel and secured. The final length of the anterior limb of the graft is determined by placing it adjacent to the humeral tunnel and visually estimating the length of the graft needed to provide adequate tension once secured in the humeral tunnel (**Figure 5,** *D*). A No. 1 braided nonabsorbable suture is placed in a Krakow fashion on the end of the anterior limb of the graft. The excess graft is excised and the graft limb is passed into the humeral tunnel with the

FIGURE 4

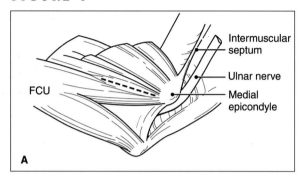

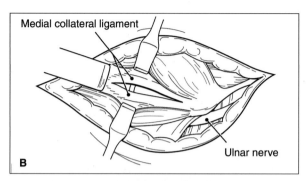

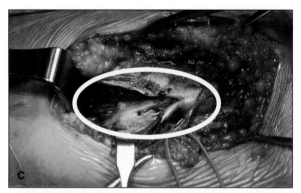

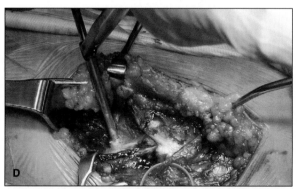

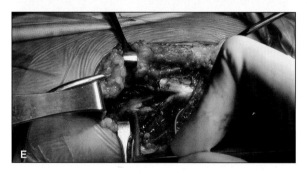

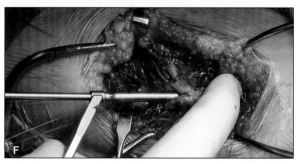

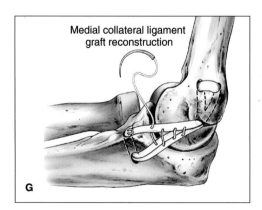

Modified Jobe technique. **A,** Drawing shows the location of the muscle split in the flexor-pronator mass. FCU = flexor carpi ulnaris. **B,** Drawing shows the muscle-splitting approach and ulnohumeral gapping demonstrated after the MCL is incised longitudinally. **C,** Intraoperative photograph demonstrates the muscle-splitting approach with MCL incision. The ulnohumeral joint, which is visible through the MCL incision, is seen inside the white oval. Intraoperative photographs show ulnar tunnels being created anterior (**D**) and posterior (**E**) to the sublime tubercle. **F,** Intraoperative photograph shows the inferior humeral tunnel being created at the anatomic MCL insertion. **G,** Drawing shows the final appearance of the original MCL reconstruction technique as described by Jobe and associates, demonstrating ulnar and humeral bone tunnels and graft figure-of-8 configuration. (Parts A and B reprinted with permission from Conway JE: The DANE TJ procedure for elbow medial ulnar collateral ligament insufficiency. *Tech Shoulder Elbow Surg* 2006;7:36-43.)

FIGURE 5

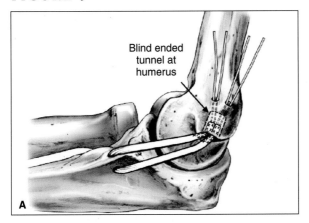

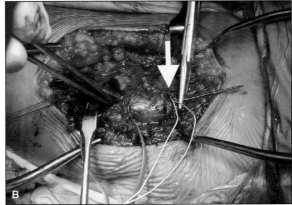

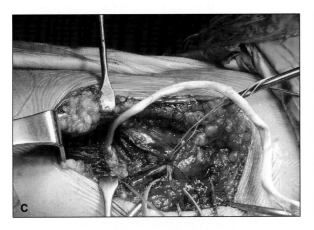

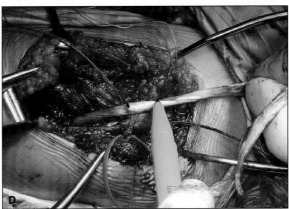

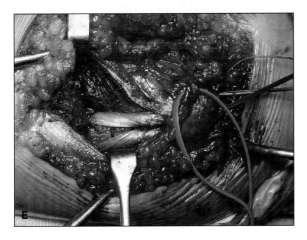

The docking technique. **A,** Drawing showing the position of the tunnels used in the docking technique. Exit holes are created superior to the inferior humeral tunnel for tensioning sutures stitched to graft. **B,** Intraoperative photograph showing sutures attached to graft being passed through humeral tunnels. **C,** Intraoperative photograph showing graft being passed through ulnar tunnels from anterior to posterior. **D,** Intraoperative photograph showing the posterior graft limb docked in the tunnel and the anterior graft limb being marked to appropriate length with marking pen. **E,** Intraoperative photograph showing final graft tensioning.

sutures exiting the small tunnels. Final graft tensioning is performed by ranging the elbow through full flexion, extension, supination, and pronation, with varus stress placed on the elbow (**Figure 5,** *E*). With the elbow in 60° of flexion and full supination, and with varus stress applied, the sutures are then tied over the bony bridge on the humeral epicondyle.

Hybrid Interference Screw Fixation Technique

Another technique of MCL reconstruction uses interference screw fixation. It achieves ulnar-sided fixation with an interference screw through a single bone tunnel and humeral fixation using the docking technique[32] (**Figure 6,** *A*). This technique has several advantages. First, it is less technically demanding because fewer drill holes are required. Second, the muscle-splitting approach used requires less dissection because only a single central ulnar tunnel is required, rather than two tunnels with an intervening bony bridge. Third, because there is no need to make a posterior ulnar tunnel, which often exits close to the ulnar nerve, morbidity to the nerve is minimized. Finally, graft passage is less difficult with an interference screw in a single tunnel. In situations in which the sublime tubercle is insufficient, such as in the case of previous fracture or prior reconstruction, the hybrid interference screw technique may be preferable.

After exposing the MCL through the muscle-splitting approach as described for the other techniques, the central isometric fiber attachments on the ulna and humeral epicondyle are identified to direct tunnel placement. At the insertion on the sublime tubercle of the ulna, approximately 4.5 mm distal to the joint surface, a 5-mm-diameter tunnel is drilled and directed 45° distally to the long axis of the ulna for a depth of 20 mm (**Figure 6,** *B*). The drill is advanced with guidance of the drill sleeve that protects the soft tissue and ulnar nerve. Maintenance of a 2-mm bone bridge from the edge of the tunnel to the joint avoids possible fracture of the tunnel into the ulnohumeral joint.

The palmaris longus tendon is harvested and folded over to create a double-strand graft. A standard whipstitch using No. 2 nonabsorbable suture is placed in the folded portion of the graft. Graft fixation into the ulnar tunnel with a 4.75 or 5.5 × 15-mm interference screw is then achieved using a unique Bio-Tenodesis driver (Arthrex, Inc, Naples, FL). The driver shaft is used to guide the turning screw into the tunnel while providing constant tension on the graft. **Figure 6,** *C* shows the graft fixed to the ulnar side and the two graft limbs ready for docking.

The humeral tunnels are created as described for the docking procedure as shown in **Figure 5,** *A*. The two limbs of the graft are then prepared as described for the docking procedure, with the modification that both limbs must be accurately cut to length. The anterior graft limb sutures are then marked with ink for later identification. One suture from the anterior graft limb and one from the posterior graft limb are then passed through the anterior humeral tunnel using a free needle or suture-passing wire. The two remaining sutures from each graft limb are passed through the posterior tunnel. The graft is delivered into the humeral tunnel and the elbow is flexed and extended with tension on the sutures to eliminate any creep. The elbow is positioned at 80° of flexion, varus stress is applied, and the posterior limb sutures are tied (**Figure 6,** *D*). Then with the elbow positioned at 30° of flexion and varus stress applied, the anterior limb sutures are tied (**Figure 6,** *E*).

Surgical Considerations

The palmaris longus is the most commonly used graft choice. All surgical candidates should be assessed for the presence of the palmaris longus because it is absent in up to 25% of the population.[33] If the palmaris longus is absent, the gracilis, Achilles, plantaris, or toe extensor tendon can be used. The gracilis generally has a predictable size and is easy to harvest. No determination can be made at this time as to which graft choice produces the best results.

The ulnar nerve also should be assessed prior to surgery. Ulnar neuritis commonly presents concurrently with MCL tears. In addition, ulnar nerve subluxation may occasionally also be present. In early reports of MCL reconstruction, the ulnar nerve was routinely transposed.[3,23] More recent technique modifications, in particular splitting the flexor-pronator origin instead of taking it down, have obviated the need for nerve transposition unless specific criteria are met. If the patient reports symptoms of ulnar neuritis (pain, numbness along the fourth and fifth digits) and nerve subluxation preoperatively, ulnar nerve transposition is indicated. Symptoms of ulnar neuritis and ulnar motor deficits

FIGURE 6

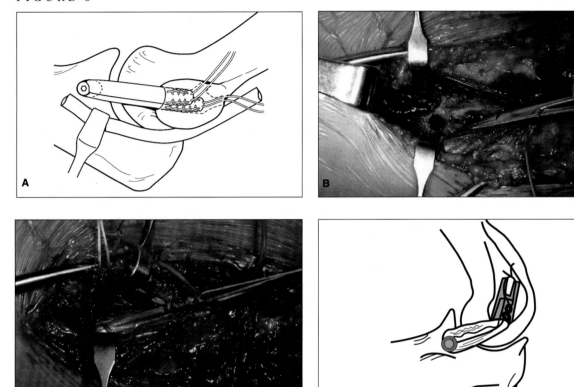

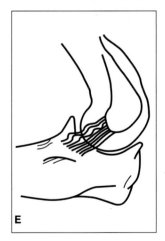

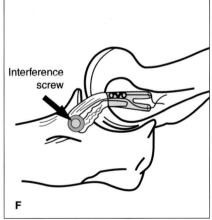

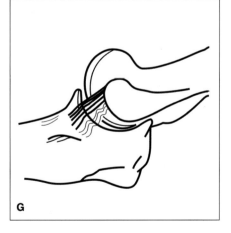

Hybrid technique of MCL reconstruction with interference screw fixation on the ulnar side and docking fixation on the humeral side. **A,** Drawing showing the completed reconstruction. **B,** Intraoperative photograph showing the ulnar tunnel for the interference screw drilled at the sublime tubercle. **C,** Intraoperative photograph showing the graft fixed in the ulna with an interference screw. Schematic illustrations demonstrate differential tensioning: in **D** and **E,** the posterior graft limb is tensioned and tied in flexion; in **F** and **G,** the anterior graft limb is tensioned and tied in extension. (Part A reprinted with permission from Conway JE: The DANE TJ procedure for elbow medial ulnar collateral ligament insufficiency. *Tech Shoulder Elbow Surg* 2006;7:36-43. Parts B and C reprinted from Ahmad CS, ElAttrache NS: Elbow valgus instability in the throwing athlete. *J Am Acad Orthop Surg* 2006;14:693-700. Parts D through G reprinted with permission from Safran M, Ahmad CS, ElAttrache NS: Ulnar collateral ligament of the elbow. *Arthroscopy* 2005;21:1381-1395.)

also are an indication for transposition. Subcutaneous transposition appears to have fewer complications than submuscular transposition.[26]

The arthroscopic valgus stress test may have some utility in assessing the competence of the MCL prior to reconstruction. In this test, the ulnohumeral joint is stressed in valgus with the forearm maximally pronated and the elbow at 90° of flexion. The ulnohumeral opening is <1 mm in most normal elbows, although this is a purely subjective observational measurement. Furthermore, a cadaveric study concluded that the anterior bundle of the MCL could not be visualized arthroscopically.[34] Indications for surgery should be based primarily on the history and physical examination. Preoperative elbow arthroscopy seems to have more of an adjunctive diagnostic utility.

Posteromedial decompression should be considered very carefully. It should not be undertaken if the patient does not have posteromedial elbow pain in extension. In addition, isolated posteromedial débridement should not be done if MCL insufficiency is present. As noted earlier, MCL resection increases valgus angulation and strain on the MCL during valgus stress. MCL insufficiency may also lead to increased posteromedial wear and subsequent osteophytes, which may result in an artificially stable joint. Therefore, isolated posteromedial decompression may render symptomatic previously asymptomatic MCL insufficiency. One series reported MCL insufficiency requiring reconstruction after isolated posteromedial decompression.[12] Azar and associates[26] and Rohrbough and associates[35] currently recommend selective minimal resection of posteromedial osteophytes in addition to MCL reconstruction.[36]

REHABILITATION

The elbow is immobilized in a splint for 10 days to allow the skin and soft tissues to heal. Sutures are removed at that time, if necessary, and active wrist, elbow, and shoulder range-of-motion exercises are initiated. After 4 to 6 weeks, strengthening exercises are begun while avoiding valgus stress until 4 months after surgery. At 4 months, the patient begins a throwing program consisting initially of ball tosses of 30 to 40 feet for about 15 minutes two to three times a week. At 5 months, the patient may increase the tossing distance to 60 feet, and at 6 months, the patient may throw lightly from the windup. At 7 months, a graduated program of range-of-motion,

strengthening, and total body conditioning exercises is undertaken. Throwers and pitchers are limited to throwing at half speed, gradually increasing the duration of the session to 25 to 30 minutes. Pitchers are permitted to throw from the pitching mound and progress to 70% of maximum velocity during the eighth or ninth month. Over the next 2 to 3 months, the duration of throwing sessions and velocity are increased incrementally to simulate a game situation. Throwing in competition is permitted at 1 year if the shoulder, elbow, and forearm are pain free while throwing and full strength and range of motion have returned. Throughout the rehabilitation phase, careful supervision and focus on body and throwing mechanics should be emphasized. Up to 18 months may be required to regain preoperative ability and competitive level with accurate ball control. Relatively shorter periods are required for other player positions or overhead sports.

OUTCOMES

Simple repair of the MCL does not yield reliable results. Most previous studies have reported better results with reconstruction than with repair.[3,23] Reported success rates after reconstruction have improved since Jobe and associates'[3] original article. In their original series, 62.5% of throwing athletes (10 of 16) returned to their preinjury level of competition. However, the original technique had a complication rate of 31.25% (5 of 16), primarily related to submuscular transposition of the ulnar nerve. Subsequently, Conway and associates[23] reported a success rate of 68% with a 95% follow-up rate. They emphasized that a history of surgery on the same elbow decreased the likelihood of an excellent result. Excluding patients with a previous operation, 74% of their patients returned to their previous level of competition. The study reported a 21% ulnar nerve complication rate. After modifying their technique further (changing flexor-pronator detachment to flexor-pronator splitting and abandoning ulnar nerve transposition in favor of no transposition), the group reported excellent results in 82% of patients, with a reduced transient ulnar nerve complication rate of 20% and no permanent ulnar nerve symptoms. Results were excellent in 93% of patients undergoing primary elbow surgery.

Results for the docking technique also have been promising. Rohrbough and associates[35] reported that 92% of their patients returned to preinjury levels of competition. Dodson and associates[37] found that 90% of their athletes undergoing MCL reconstruction using the docking technique returned to the same or a higher level of competitive throwing. Recently, in a 2-year follow-up study, Paletta and associates[38] reported that 92% of elite baseball players (23 of 25) were able to return to preinjury levels of competition using the docking technique. They reported a mean time to return of 11.5 months and only two complications.

Interference screw fixation is a newer technique that has potential advantages. Ahmad and associates[39] conducted a biomechanical cadaveric study demonstrating that a technique using interference screw fixation on both the ulna and the humerus restored valgus stability at all flexion angles and achieved strength of fixation to a level approaching that of an intact ligament. McAdams and associates[40] compared cyclic valgus loading on reconstructions using the bioabsorbable interference screw procedure and docking procedure using cadaver elbows. The interference screw fixation resulted in less valgus angulation in response to early cyclic valgus load as compared with the docking technique.

Dines and associates[41] reported the results of an initial series of 22 patients treated with the hybrid interference screw technique that has been referred to as the DANE TJ technique. At 36 months' follow-up, 19 of 22 patients had excellent results, 2 had fair results, and there was 1 poor result, which was a revision case. The two other revision MCL reconstructions had excellent outcomes. When used in two cases of sublime tubercle avulsions, the results were excellent.

In contrast, a recent cadaveric study compared four different reconstruction methods with respect to initial fixation strength when subjected to initial peak loads and repeated valgus loading.[42] The study evaluated the figure-of-8, docking, single-strand interference screw, and EndoButton (Smith & Nephew, Memphis, TN) techniques. The authors concluded that all reconstructions had a lower peak load to failure than the intact ligament. Furthermore, the docking and EndoButton techniques had higher peak and cyclical loading characteristics than the figure-of-8 and single-strand interference screw techniques. Large and associates[43] performed a biomechanical cadaveric study comparing the strength provided by the Jobe technique and the interference screw technique with that of intact MCL. They found that, compared with the interference screw technique, the Jobe bone tunnel technique created a much stronger construct that more closely approximated the tensile properties of the intact native MCL. In general, the bone tunnel technique failed with tunnel breakage, while the interference screw technique failed with graft slippage. Long-term follow-up of these new techniques in the clinical setting has not yet been reported.

CONCLUSIONS

MCL reconstruction is a technically demanding procedure. The surgeon must work to perfect several factors, including graft isometry, tension, and security, while optimizing the healing environment. In properly selected patients, MCL reconstruction can be successful in returning elite athletes to their preinjury level of play. Excellent results are generally achieved with a flexor-pronator muscle-splitting approach without ulnar nerve transposition (unless indicated), using a figure-of-8 or docking technique. Transient ulnar nerve symptoms are common. Judicious concurrent posteromedial osteophyte excision may be performed if required. A history of prior elbow surgery diminishes the likelihood of an excellent result. A number of new techniques, including interference screw fixation, have yet to be validated in the clinical setting.

REFERENCES

1. Morrey BF, An KN: Articular and ligamentous contributions to the stability of the elbow joint. *Am J Sports Med* 1983;11:315-319.

2. Waris W: Elbow injuries in javelin throwers. *Acta Chir Scand* 1946;93:563.

3. Jobe FW, Stark H, Lombardo SJ: Reconstruction of the ulnar collateral ligament in athletes. *J Bone Joint Surg Am* 1986;68:1158-1163.

4. Cain EL Jr, Dugas JR, Wolf RS, Andrews JR: Elbow injuries in throwing athletes: A current concepts review. *Am J Sports Med* 2003;31:621-635.

5. Morrey BF, Tanaka S, An KN: Valgus stability of the elbow: A definition of primary and secondary constraints. *Clin Orthop Relat Res* 1991;265:187-195.

6. Callaway GH, Field LD, Deng XH, et al: Biomechanical evaluation of the medial collateral ligament of the elbow. *J Bone Joint Surg Am* 1997;79:1223-1231.

7. Fleisig GS, Andrews JR, Dillman CJ, Escamilla RF: Kinetics of baseball pitching with implications about injury mechanisms. *Am J Sports Med* 1995;23:233-239.

8. Werner SL, Fleisig GS, Dillman CJ, Andrews JR: Biomechanics of the elbow during baseball pitching. *J Orthop Sports Phys Ther* 1993;17:274-278.

9. Elliott B, Fleisig G, Nicholls R, Escamilia R: Technique effects on upper limb loading in the tennis serve. *J Sci Med Sport* 2003;6:76-87.

10. Fleisig G, Nicholls R, Elliott B, Escamilla R: Kinematics used by world class tennis players to produce high-velocity serves. *Sports Biomech* 2003;2:51-64.

11. Park MC, Ahmad CS: Dynamic contributions of the flexor-pronator mass to elbow valgus stability. *J Bone Joint Surg Am* 2004;86:2268-2274.

12. Andrews JR, Timmerman LA: Outcome of elbow surgery in professional baseball players. *Am J Sports Med* 1995;23:407-413.

13. Kamineni S, Hirahara H, Pomianowski S, et al: Partial posteromedial olecranon resection: A kinematic study. *J Bone Joint Surg Am* 2003;85:1005-1011.

14. Kamineni S, ElAttrache NS, O'Driscoll SW, et al: Medial collateral ligament strain with partial posteromedial olecranon resection: A biomechanical study. *J Bone Joint Surg Am* 2004;86:2424-2430.

15. Ahmad CS, Park MC, Elattrache NS: Elbow medial ulnar collateral ligament insufficiency alters posteromedial olecranon contact. *Am J Sports Med* 2004;32:1607-1612.

16. Safran M, Ahmad CS, Elattrache NS: Ulnar collateral ligament of the elbow. *Arthroscopy* 2005;21:1381-1395.

17. Thompson WH, Jobe FW, Yocum LA, Pink MM: Ulnar collateral ligament reconstruction in athletes: Muscle-splitting approach without transposition of the ulnar nerve. *J Shoulder Elbow Surg* 2001;10:152-157.

18. Veltri DM, O'Brien SJ, Field LD, et al: The milking maneuver: A new test to evaluate the MCL of the elbow in the throwing athlete. 10th Open Meeting of the American Shoulder and Elbow Surgeons Specialty Day, New Orleans, LA, 1994.

19. Ellenbecker TS, Mattalino AJ, Elam EA, Caplinger RA: Medial elbow joint laxity in professional baseball pitchers: A bilateral comparison using stress radiography. *Am J Sports Med* 1998;26:420-424.

20. O'Driscoll SW, Lawton RL, Smith AM: The "moving valgus stress test" for medial collateral ligament tears of the elbow. *Am J Sports Med* 2005;33:231-239.

21. Safran MR, McGarry MH, Shin S, Han S, Lee TQ: Effects of elbow flexion and forearm rotation on valgus laxity of the elbow. *J Bone Joint Surg Am* 2005;87:2065-2074.

22. Norwood LA, Shook JA, Andrews JR: Acute medial elbow ruptures. *Am J Sports Med* 1981;9:16-19.

23. Conway JE, Jobe FW, Glousman RE, Pink M: Medial instability of the elbow in throwing athletes: Treatment by repair or reconstruction of the ulnar collateral ligament. *J Bone Joint Surg Am* 1992;74:67-83.

24. Rijke AM, Goitz HT, McCue FC, Andrews JR, Berr SS: Stress radiography of the medial elbow ligaments. *Radiology* 1994;191:213-216.

25. Conway J: Abstract: Secondary effects of ulnar collateral ligament injury. Clinical, radiographic and arthroscopic perspective, in *Book of Abstracts and Outlines*. Rosemont, IL, American Orthopaedic Society for Sports Medicine, 1999, pp 356-357.

26. Azar FM, Andrews JR, Wilk KE, Groh D: Operative treatment of ulnar collateral ligament injuries of the elbow in athletes. *Am J Sports Med* 2000;28:16-23.

27. Timmerman LA, Schwartz ML, Andrews JR: Preoperative evaluation of the ulnar collateral ligament by magnetic resonance imaging and computed tomography arthrography: Evaluation in 25 baseball players with surgical confirmation. *Am J Sports Med* 1994;22:26-31.

28. Munshi M, Pretterklieber ML, Chung CB, et al: Anterior bundle of ulnar collateral ligament: Evaluation of anatomic relationships by using MR imaging, MR arthrography, and gross anatomic and histologic analysis. *Radiology* 2004;231:797-803.

29. Sasaki J, Takahara M, Ogino T, Kashiwa H, Ishigaki D, Kanauchi Y: Ultrasonographic assessment of the ulnar collateral ligament and medial elbow laxity in college baseball players. *J Bone Joint Surg Am* 2002;84:525-531.

30. Nazarian LN, McShane JM, Ciccotti MG, O'Kane PL, Harwood MI: Dynamic US of the anterior band of the ulnar collateral ligament of the elbow in asymptomatic major league baseball pitchers. *Radiology* 2003;227:149-154.

31. Rettig AC, Sherrill C, Snead DS, Mendler JC, Mieling P: Nonoperative treatment of ulnar collateral ligament injuries in throwing athletes. *Am J Sports Med* 2001;29:15-17.

32. Conway JE: The DANE TJ procedure for elbow medial ulnar collateral ligament insufficiency. *Tech Shoulder Elbow Surg* 2006;7:36-43.

33. Thompson NW, Mockford BJ, Cran GW: Absence of the palmaris longus muscle: A population study. *Ulster Med J* 2001;70:22-24.

34. Field LD, Callaway GH, O'Brien SJ, Altchek DW: Arthroscopic assessment of the medial collateral ligament complex of the elbow. *Am J Sports Med* 1995;23:396-400.

35. Rohrbough JT, Altchek DW, Hyman J, Williams RJ III, Botts JD: Medial collateral ligament reconstruction of the elbow using the docking technique. *Am J Sports Med* 2002;30:541-548.

36. Purcell DB, Matava MJ, Wright RW: Ulnar collateral ligament reconstruction: A systematic review. *Clin Orthop Relat Res* 2007;455:72-77.

37. Dodson CC, Thomas A, Dines JS, Nho SJ, Williams RJ III, Altchek DW: Medial ulnar collateral ligament reconstruction of the elbow in throwing athletes. *Am J Sports Med* 2006;34:1926-1932.

38. Paletta GA Jr, Wright RW: The modified docking procedure for elbow ulnar collateral ligament reconstruction: 2-year follow-up in elite throwers. *Am J Sports Med* 2006;34:1594-1598.

39. Ahmad CS, Lee TQ, ElAttrache NS: Biomechanical evaluation of a new ulnar collateral ligament reconstruction technique with interference screw fixation. *Am J Sports Med* 2003;31:332-337.

40. McAdams TR, Lee AT, Centeno J, Giori NJ, Lindsey DP: Two ulnar collateral ligament reconstruction methods: The docking technique versus bioabsorbable interference screw fixation. A biomechanical evaluation with cyclic loading. *J Shoulder Elbow Surg* 2007;16:224-228.

41. Dines JS, ElAttrache NS, Conway JE, Smith W, Ahmad CS: Clinical outcomes of the DANE TJ technique to treat ulnar collateral ligament insufficiency of the elbow. *Am J Sports Med* 2007;35:2039-2044.

42. Armstrong AD, Dunning CE, Ferreira LM, Faber KJ, Johnson JA, King GJ: A biomechanical comparison of four reconstruction techniques for the medial collateral ligament-deficient elbow. *J Shoulder Elbow Surg* 2005;14:207-215.

43. Large TM, Coley ER, Peindl RD, Fleischli JE: A biomechanical comparison of 2 ulnar collateral ligament reconstruction techniques. *Arthroscopy* 2007;23:141-150.

CHAPTER 6

POSTEROLATERAL ROTATORY INSTABILITY OF THE ELBOW AND LATERAL ULNAR COLLATERAL LIGAMENT RECONSTRUCTION

CHRISTOPHER S. AHMAD, MD
DEREK MOORE, MD
JOHN E. CONWAY, MD

Posterolateral rotatory instability of the elbow was first described in 1991. Since then, tremendous research has further elucidated the anatomy and pathophysiology of this instability pattern. The essential lesion is disruption of the lateral collateral ligament complex. Recent improvements have been made in diagnostic physical examination maneuvers and surgical reconstruction techniques.

ANATOMY

The lateral collateral ligament complex of the elbow can be anatomically and functionally divided into the radial collateral ligament (RCL), the lateral ulnar collateral ligament (LUCL), the annular ligament, and the accessory lateral collateral ligament (**Figure 1**). The ligament complex lies beneath the fascia covering the supinator and the extensor carpi ulnaris muscles. The LUCL originates on the lateral epicondyle and inserts on the supinator crest of the ulna,[1,2] which is the bony prominence just distal and posterior to the radial head on the ulna. The origin of the lateral collateral ligament complex lies near the elbow axis of rotation, so it is relatively isometric throughout elbow range of motion.[1] The RCL originates on the lateral epicondyle and inserts onto the annular ligament. This ligament has an average length of 20 mm and width of 8 mm. The annular ligament surrounds the radial head and stabilizes the proximal radioulnar joint. The accessory lateral collateral ligament stabilizes the annular ligament by connecting it to the supinator crest.

PATHOPHYSIOLOGY

The LUCL has been established as the primary stabilizer of posterolateral rotational stability in the elbow.[2,3] Posterolateral rotatory instability (PLRI) of the elbow can result from traumatic elbow subluxation, dislocation, or iatrogenic injury to the lateral ligament complex during lateral elbow surgery (eg, treatment of lateral epicondylitis). The instability allows the radial head to either subluxate or dislocate posteriorly when the elbow is positioned in slight flexion, forearm supination, and valgus stress.[3-5]

During posterolateral rotation, the proximal forearm rotates so that the coronoid passes under the trochlea as the radial head moves posterior to the capitellum. PLRI is considered the first phase of elbow instability that can progress to frank dislocation. The soft-tissue injuries are sequential, with disruption beginning laterally and progressing medially. First injured are the LUCL and RCL, with a PLRI pattern that typically reduces spontaneously. Progression of the injury causes disruption of the anterior and posterior capsule, which allows

FIGURE 1

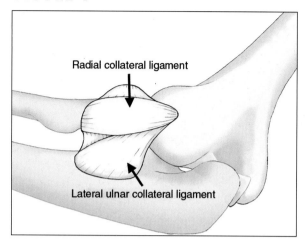

The lateral collateral ligament complex of the elbow.

ulnohumeral subluxation. Complete dislocation may also disrupt the medial collateral ligament complex, but medial ligament injury is not required for elbow dislocation to occur.

Mechanism of Injury

PLRI commonly occurs in patients with a history of an elbow dislocation; however, some may have experienced recurrent elbow subluxations. The injury results from a combination of axial compression, external rotation (supination), and valgus forces applied to the elbow as a result of a fall onto an outstretched arm. PLRI is also seen as a complication after lateral surgical approaches to the elbow, especially for lateral epicondylitis surgery. In addition, PLRI may occur after surgery using the Kocher approach for radial head fractures if the lateral collateral ligament complex, which is often violated by the Kocher approach, is not repaired meticulously.

CLINICAL EVALUATION

A history of trauma to the elbow usually precedes symptoms of painful clicking or locking of the elbow, which occur with the elbow under axial load in a position of slight flexion with the forearm in supination.[3,5,6] An elbow dislocation may be the initial event, especially in patients younger than 20 years of age. In older patients, varus extension stress without true dislocation is more common.[5] A history of prior surgery to the elbow that may have injured the LUCL must also be sought on history.

Examination maneuvers to demonstrate PLRI have been challenging. Several physical examination tests have been described to identify PLRI—the posterolateral rotatory apprehension test, or lateral pivot-shift test; the posterolateral rotatory drawer test; the stand-up test; and the push-up test. The posterolateral rotatory apprehension test is performed with the patient supine and the affected extremity overhead. The elbow is supinated and a valgus moment and axial load is applied while the elbow is flexed, as shown in **Figure 2**, *A*. The maneuver produces apprehension and reproduction of the patient's symptoms. The actual subluxation and the clunk that occurs with reduction may not be appreciated without local or general anesthesia. When observed, the actual pivot shift appears as a radial head prominence and formation of a dimple between the radial head and the capitellum (**Figure 2**, *B* through *D*). As the elbow is flexed >40°, reduction of the ulna and radius occurs with a palpable and visual clunk.

The elbow posterolateral rotatory drawer test is performed with the patient supine and the arm overhead with the elbow flexed 40° to 90°. Similar to a Lachman examination for the knee, the humerus is stabilized and the ulna and radius are translated away from the humerus posterolaterally, pivoting around the intact medial ulnar collateral ligament. In the stand-up test, the patient attempts to stand up from a seated position by pushing on the seat with the elbow fully supinated. Reproduction of the patient's symptoms indicates a positive test. A similar push-up test is performed by having the patient attempt a push-up from the prone position with the forearms maximally supinated, and then again with the forearms maximally pronated. The test is positive if symptoms occur with the forearms supinated, but not pronated.

Standard radiographs are most often normal, but degenerative changes may be seen with chronic PLRI. Fluoroscopy or a lateral stress radiograph at the point of maximum rotatory subluxation during the pivot-shift test before feeling the clunk can demonstrate the rotatory subluxation and confirms the diagnosis. Finally, MRI is becoming more useful to assist in the diagnosis.

Although arthroscopy cannot accurately diagnose PLRI, arthroscopic maneuvers may suggest PLRI. The pivot-shift test is performed while viewing from the anteromedial portal. The radial head will rotate and

FIGURE 2

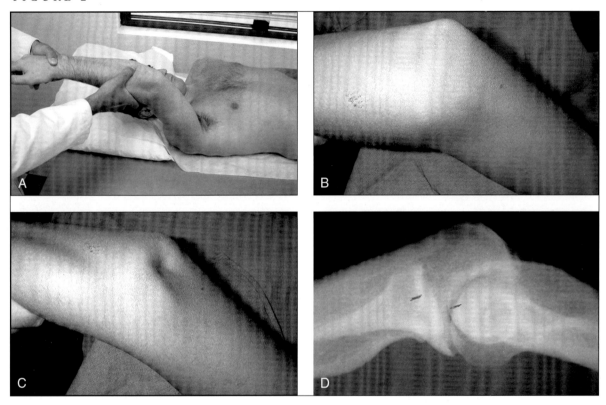

The posterolateral rotatory apprehension test, or lateral pivot-shift test. **A,** Valgus, supination, and axial forces are applied. **B,** The radial head is reduced. **C,** The radial head subluxated posteriorly with pivot-shift examination, causing a dimple to appear. **D,** Lateral radiograph demonstrating posterior subluxation of the radial head. (Parts B-D reproduced with permission from Conway JC, Singleton SB: Posterolateral rotatory instability of the elbow. *Sports Med Arthrosc Rev* 2003;11;71-78.)

translate posteriorly if PLRI is present. In addition, the lateral drive-through sign, in which the arthroscope is easily driven through the lateral gutter and into the lateral aspect of the ulnohumeral joint, is present in PLRI.

INDICATIONS FOR RECONSTRUCTION

Lateral complex reconstruction is indicated in patients with history, physical examination, and imaging studies consistent with chronic symptomatic PLRI. PLRI of the elbow, especially of a moderate to severe degree, warrants LUCL reconstruction in addition to native ligament repair. The goal is to stabilize the elbow and avoid complications such as restricting range of motion. Relative contraindications include skeletal immaturity, neuropathic joints (Charcot arthritis), and patients who are

unwilling or unable to comply with postoperative rehabilitation. Repair, rather than reconstruction, should be considered in skeletally immature patients and in acute injuries when adequate tissue is available. The presence of coexisting injuries to the joint, such as fractures and osteochondral injuries, should also be addressed as indicated.

SURGICAL TECHNIQUE

Surgical techniques described have included radial collateral and annular ligament repair,[6] reconstruction with biceps and triceps tendon slips to the olecranon and coronoid process,[7] and extra-articular bone block to the coronoid process and/or the olecranon fossa.[8] The most successful surgical techniques reconstruct the lateral ligament complex. Nestor and associates[5] described a lig-

FIGURE 3

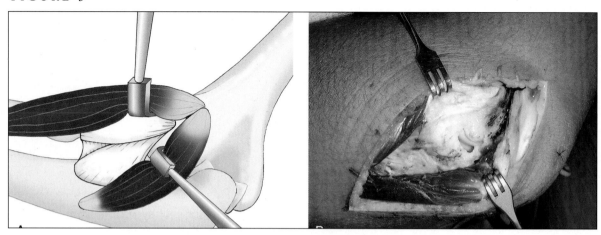

Drawing **(A)** and intraoperative photograph **(B)** demonstrating the Kocher approach to expose the supinator crest and lateral epicondyle.

ament reconstruction using palmaris longus tendon graft and bone tunnels on the ulna and humerus. Refinement of the technique now includes a "yoke stitch" to improve graft tensioning,[9] making the ulnar tunnels perpendicular to the LUCL and proximal humeral tunnels anterior to the supracondylar ridge.[10]

A technique of hybrid fixation for LUCL reconstruction has been developed based on its success for reconstructing the medial ulnar collateral ligament, employing interference screw fixation on the ulna and docking fixation on the epicondyle.[11] This technique has been used clinically but results have not been reported. Graft choices include the gracilis tendon, the palmaris longus tendon, the fourth toe extensor tendon, the plantaris tendon, a 3-mm-wide strip of the Achilles tendon, and numerous allograft tissues. Patients being considered should be assessed for the presence of the palmaris longus tendon.[12] Our preference is the ipsilateral gracilis tendon because of its consistent size and presence.

Patient Positioning

The patient is positioned supine, and general or regional anesthesia is established. Examination under anesthesia is performed to confirm the diagnosis of a PLRI with the lateral pivot-shift test (**Figure 2**). Fluoroscopy during the maneuver may further document and confirm the instability. A tourniquet is placed on the upper arm and the ipsilateral thigh (if gracilis graft is chosen) and both the upper and lower extremities are prepared and

draped. Gracilis or palmaris longus graft harvest is performed.

Approach

After exsanguination and tourniquet inflation, the arm is held across the chest. Either a 15-cm direct posterior elbow incision or direct incision from the lateral epicondyle curving just posterior to the radial head toward the lateral ulna is used. A lateral flap is raised, and the interval between the extensor carpi ulnaris and anconeus is developed. The supinator crest and the anatomic attachment of the LUCL is exposed (**Figure 3**).

O'Driscoll LUCL Reconstruction

The technique of LUCL reconstruction described by O'Driscoll creates tunnels on the ulna at the supinator crest and lateral epicondyle, with a graft woven through the tunnels (**Figure 4**). The redundant lateral capsule is incised from the radial head to the lateral epicondyle in line with the fibers of the LUCL. Two 3.2-mm holes are drilled on the proximal and distal portion of the supinator crest with a minimum 5-mm bone bridge. The supinator crest is a palpable tubercle just distal to the annular ligament attachment. The tunnels are connected using an angled curet. The isometric point of insertion onto the lateral epicondyle is determined by passing a suture through the ulnar tunnels and positioning the sutures over the epicondyle while moving the elbow

FIGURE 4

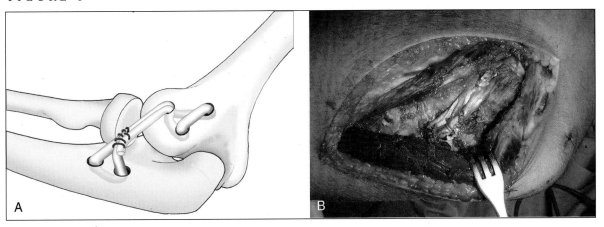

Drawing (**A**) and intraoperative photograph (**B**) demonstrating tunnel location, graft placement, and graft fixation in the O'Driscoll technique.

through flexion and extension. The initial humeral tunnel is created with a 4-mm drill at the isometric point and directed proximally. This tunnel is connected to two angled tunnels created proximally with a 3.2-mm drill. The tunnels are connected with angled curets. The graft is passed through the ulnar tunnels and fixed by suturing the graft limbs together. The free limb of the graft is then passed through the humeral tunnels. With the elbow positioned in 40° of flexion and the forearm fully pronated, the graft limbs are sutured together for graft fixation. The capsule is closed and imbricated. The muscle split is closed, the skin is closed, and a splint is applied with the elbow pronated and in 90° of flexion.

Interference Screw Hybrid Technique

The interference screw hybrid technique (**Figure 5**) is designed to achieve an anatomic reconstruction of the lateral collateral ligament complex. Although this technique has been used clinically, no results have yet been reported. The same Kocher approach as described above is employed. The RCL and LUCL are released from the humeral epicondyle, and the RCL is then divided from the LUCL. Graft preparation for a gracilis or palmaris longus tendon is performed. After stripping muscle from the tendon, the tendon is folded in half to create a double-strand graft and a locking Krackow suture using No. 2 FiberWire (Arthrex Inc, Naples, FL) is placed in the folded end for a distance of 20 mm. The folded end of the graft is then sized to determine the ulnar tunnel diameter, which is typically 5 mm.

Following this, a 2.7-mm pin is placed at the anatomic insertion of the LUCL on the supinator crest. A tunnel is drilled with a diameter 1 mm larger than the graft diameter and to a depth of approximately 20 mm (**Figure 5**, *A*). The tendon graft is delivered into the ulnar tunnel using the Bio-Tenodesis driver (Arthrex) and fixed with an interference screw sized to be the same or slightly smaller than the tunnel diameter. The screw is positioned on the driver with the driver thumb pad fully retracted to the handle. The free ends of a looped No. 2 FiberWire are then passed through the cannulation of the driver. The graft sutures and the graft are passed through the suture loop. As the suture loop is withdrawn through the driver, the graft is positioned to allow the loop to capture the graft at the tip of the driver. With the graft connected to the tip of the driver, the driver tip and graft are delivered into the bone tunnel. The driver then provides constant tension of the graft onto the tunnel while the screw is advanced into the tunnel. If the interference fit is too tight, which is appreciated by difficulty advancing the screw, the tunnel should be drilled to a slightly larger diameter. Forcing the screw without expanding the tunnel may cause injury to the graft. The paired sutures, one woven into the graft and outside the screw and one looped over the graft and passed through the cannulation in the screw, are then tied, locking the graft to the interference screw. This creates combined interference screw fixation and suture anchor–type fixation. For fixation to fail, either the sutures must break with the graft slipping past the screw,

FIGURE 5

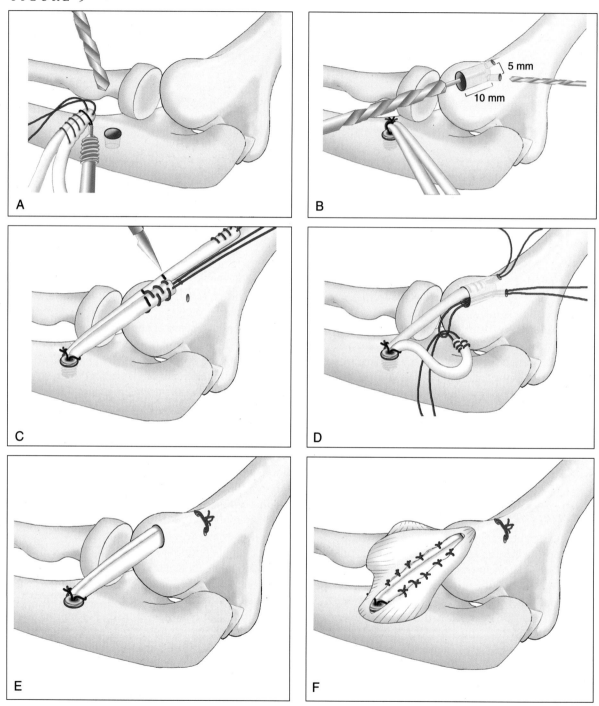

Interference screw hybrid technique. **A,** Ulnar tunnel created with interference screw graft fixation. **B,** Epicondyle tunnel created with exit tunnels. **C,** Graft is measured to accurate length. **D,** Graft is passed into docking tunnel. **E,** Graft is passed and docked into the humeral epicondyle tunnel. **F,** Native LUCL and capsule are imbricated, demonstrating final reconstruction.

or the graft and screw must pull out together. Ahmad and associates[13] evaluated the fixation for medial ulnar collateral ligament reconstruction and found that the failure strength was 90% of the native ligament.

Another advantage of locking the graft to the screw is that the increased fixation strength allows use of smaller diameter screws to reduce graft trauma. Depending on the density of the bone, enlarging the tunnel opening by 0.5 mm may ease graft and screw placement and decrease trauma to the graft from the interference screw. Attention is then turned to humeral tunnel creation.

Humeral tunnel position is checked for isometry by holding the graft over the epicondyle and flexing and extending the elbow. A guide pin is placed in the lateral epicondyle at the isometric point, which is slightly anterior to the inferiormost aspect of the epicondyle. A unicortical tunnel the same diameter as the graft is created to a length of approximately 15 mm. Exit holes of 2.5 mm are drilled from the proximal aspect of the epicondyle into that initial tunnel, separated by an 8-mm bony bridge (**Figure 5,** *B*). Each of the two limbs of the graft is measured against the epicondyle and marked as shown in **Figure 5,** *C*. Each limb is then sutured with a No. 2 nonabsorbable FiberWire suture in a Krackow suture fashion and excess graft is removed.

The native RCL is controlled with a No. 0 nonabsorbable suture placed in a Krackow fashion. The sutures are then passed with the graft sutures into the epicondyle exit tunnels (**Figure 5,** *D* and *E*). While the graft tension is maintained, the radiohumeral and ulnohumeral articulations are verified to be stable with supination, extension, and valgus stress to the elbow. Graft position is verified to be isometric for a full range of elbow motion. The sutures are tied over the bone bridge with the elbow in 30° to 40° of flexion and the forearm pronated. Finally, the capsule, including the redundant RCL and the LUCL, are imbricated into the soft-tissue reconstruction using No. 0 nonabsorbable suture (**Figure 5,** *F*). Full range of motion is confirmed and, by using fluoroscopy and physical examination, elbow stability is verified. The muscle fascia is closed and the skin is closed routinely. The elbow is then splinted in 90° of flexion.

REHABILITATION

The reconstruction is protected by immobilizing the elbow in 90° of flexion and full pronation for a period of 2 weeks. This is followed by use of a hinged brace for a period of 4 to 6 weeks depending on the strength of the repair, coexisting morbidities, and patient compliance. The patient is allowed to begin immediate pronation/supination with the elbow flexed 90° or greater. Routine activities are permitted at 3 months, and strenuous activities are avoided until 6 months postoperatively.

OUTCOMES

O'Driscoll and associates[14] suggested that if there is no degenerative arthritis and the radial head is intact, then approximately 90% of patients have a satisfactory outcome. If the radial head is excised or there is degenerative arthritis of the humeroulnar joint, there is only a 67% to 75% satisfactory outcome. LUCL reconstruction is technically demanding with regard to achieving graft isometry and graft fixation. Sanchez-Sotelo and associates[9] reported that in 90% of patients, stability was restored following LUCL reconstruction and excellent results achieved in only approximately 60% of patients.

The technique of interference screw fixation has been biomechanically evaluated in cadavers, and graft fixation strength was 90% that of control intact medial ulnar collateral ligaments under valgus load.[13] However, clinical follow-up data have not yet been presented for the new hybrid interference screw technique.

REFERENCES

1. Morrey BF, An KN: Functional anatomy of the ligaments of the elbow. *Clin Orthop Relat Res* 1985;201: 84-90.

2. O'Driscoll SW, Horii E, Morrey BF, Carmichael SW: Anatomy of the ulnar part of the lateral collateral ligament of the elbow. *Clin Anat* 1992;5:296-303.

3. O'Driscoll SW, Bell DF, Morrey BF: Posterolateral rotatory instability of the elbow. *J Bone Joint Surg Am* 1991;73:440-446.

4. Cohen MS, Hastings H II: Rotatory instability of the elbow: The anatomy and role of the lateral stabilizers. *J Bone Joint Surg Am* 1997;79:225-233.

5. Nestor BJ, O'Driscoll SW, Morrey BF: Ligamentous reconstruction for posterolateral rotatory instability of the elbow. *J Bone Joint Surg Am* 1992;74:1235-1241.

6. Osborne G, Cotterill P: Recurrent dislocation of the elbow. *J Bone Joint Surg Br* 1966;48:340-346.

7. Kapel O: Operation for habitual dislocation of the elbow. *J Bone Joint Surg Am* 1951;33:707-710.

8. Milch H: Bilateral recurrent dislocation of the ulna at the elbow. *J Bone Joint Surg Am* 1936;18:777-780.

9. Sanchez-Sotelo J, Morrey BF, O'Driscoll SW: Ligamentous repair and reconstruction for posterolateral rotatory instability of the elbow. *J Bone Joint Surg Br* 2005;87:54-61.

10. O'Driscoll SW, Morrey BF: *Surgical Reconstruction of the Lateral Collateral Ligament*, ed 2. Philadelphia, PA, Lippincott Williams & Wilkins, 2002.

11. Conway JE: The DANE TJ procedure for elbow medial ulnar collateral ligament insufficiency. *Tech Shoulder Elbow Surg* 2006;7:36-43.

12. Vanderhooft E: The frequency of and relationship between the palmaris longus and plantaris tendons. *Am J Orthop* 1996;25:38-41.

13. Ahmad CS, Lee TQ, ElAttrache NS: Biomechanical evaluation of a new ulnar collateral ligament reconstruction technique with interference screw fixation. *Am J Sports Med* 2003;31:332-337.

14. O'Driscoll SW, Jupiter JB, King GJ, Hotchkiss RN, Morrey BF: The unstable elbow. *Instr Course Lect* 2001;50:89-102.

CHAPTER 7

VALGUS EXTENSION OVERLOAD AND PLICA

SHAWN W. O'DRISCOLL, PHD, MD

BACKGROUND AND RELEVANT BIOMECHANICS

Valgus extension overload (VEO), or chronic valgus overload, is not a diagnosis but rather a term given to an array of conditions commonly affecting the dominant elbow in overhead athletes. The spectrum of chronic injuries and their sequelae includes injuries to the medial collateral ligament (MCL), valgus instability, flexor-pronator tendinopathies, ulnar neuritis, posteromedial trochlear chondral erosion, posteromedial impingement, olecranon stress fractures, and lateral joint compartment problems such as osteochondritis dissecans and radiocapitellar arthritis.

Disabilities in overhead athletes—baseball pitchers and catchers, javelin throwers, and others—have been recognized for decades. The pathologies, potential etiologies, and prognoses have been discussed and refined from the early reports by Bennett,[1] Waris,[2] Slocum,[3] and King and associates.[4] The pitching motion, which can be thought of as a model for other overhead activity sports, is typically divided into the windup, cocking, acceleration, deceleration, and follow-through phases.[5-9] Valgus torque peaks at potentially injurious levels around 35 N·m during the late cocking and acceleration phases as the internal rotators of the shoulder initiate humeral internal rotation. These approximate the MCL failure load of 35 ± 10 N·m, proving that muscular stabilization is required to protect the MCL. During deceleration, elbow compressive forces of 850 to 1,100 N and 450 to 650 N (approximately body weight) have been reported for pitching and football throws, respectively. The combination of torques and

forces causes repetitive tensile stresses medially, compressive stresses laterally, and impaction/shear stresses posteriorly. The final common pathway is hypertrophic degenerative arthritis similar to that seen in other repetitive overuse situations (weightlifting, production line work activity, etc) affecting the elbow. The main difference in overhead athletes relates to the distribution of arthritic changes (osteophytes and articular injuries) during the early stages of degeneration.

CLINICAL PRESENTATION

VEO presents several different ways. The most common is medial elbow pain, but the pain can be posterior or lateral, depending on the primary pathology. VEO in throwing athletes commonly presents with pain and declining performance in the form of decreased endurance, accuracy, and velocity. Medial elbow pain in a thrower is always concerning for ligamentous injury, but other structures can be injured in isolation or association with ligamentous injury and should be examined closely to establish the true cause of the patient's pain. In fact, even patients undergoing surgical reconstruction for chronic injury to the MCL may have associated pathologies requiring treatment. Tendinitis of the common flexor-pronator origin, medial triceps muscle subluxation, ulnar nerve irritation, and chondral or osteochondral defects[10] in the posteromedial trochlea, as well as local stress fractures,[11,12] all are possible causes of medial elbow pain in throwers and may exist alone or in association with the other causes of pain.

Careful history and physical examination are usually sufficient for either the establishment of an accurate diagnosis or the prediction that such will be confirmed with further investigation. The athlete should be questioned about the effect of the injury on performance and the onset of the pain (sudden or long-standing). Factors such as the quality, location, and timing of the pain are important historical factors that should be elicited. A comprehensive elbow examination should be conducted, including an assessment of tenderness to palpation of precise anatomic locations (medial triceps, ulnar nerve, MCL, medial epicondyle, common flexor origin, etc). Range of motion, strength, stability, and neurologic status should be carefully evaluated for each patient, along with provocative tests that have been developed for each specific diagnosis.

MEDIAL COLLATERAL LIGAMENT INJURY

MCL injury is one of the more common problems affecting the elbow of overhead athletes and frequently presents as a spectrum of injury. Acute injuries due to spontaneous failure of the ligamentous complex may present after a "popping" sensation. However, many athletes present with a vague onset of medial elbow pain associated with inability to perform at 100% effort (decreased accuracy, velocity, endurance).[13-17] The source of this more chronic elbow pain usually involves attenuation or partial tearing of the deep anterior bundle of the MCL, leading to "chronic valgus extension overload" syndrome with traumatic or degenerative arthritis of the elbow, capitellar wear, posteromedial osteophytes, flexion contractures, and ulnar nerve symptoms.[18,19] Although the acute, complete tears are more straightforward to diagnose, partial tears and ligament attenuation often present a considerable diagnostic challenge.[20,21]

Static imaging studies are rarely diagnostic, and the role of stress radiographs in the diagnosis of medial elbow ligamentous insufficiency can be confusing and even misleading when attempting to manage a throwing athlete.[22,23] Although the contralateral elbow may serve as an appropriate control in normal volunteers, recent evidence suggests that this may not be true in throwing athletes. Ellenbecker and associates[24] performed stress radiographs on bilateral elbows of 40 asymptomatic baseball pitchers and found a significantly larger medial ulnohumeral opening in the throwing arm compared to the nonthrowing arm, suggesting an acquired medial laxity.

Despite the ready availability of sophisticated imaging studies such as MRI, CT arthrography, and ultrasonography, diagnostic accuracy has been at best inconsistent.[25-29] Arthroscopic valgus stress testing has also been routinely used to assess elbow ligamentous stability. Timmerman and Andrews[30,31] described seven patients with persistent medial elbow pain when throwing; six of the seven athletes had normal MRI examinations, with all patients demonstrating a positive arthroscopic valgus stress test and surgically confirmed partial tears of the MCL. Field and Altchek[32] examined cadaveric elbows via arthroscopy with sequential release of the MCL and demonstrated that the entire anterior bundle of the MCL had to be released before significant medial ulnohumeral opening could be identified, which raises concerns about the appropriate identification of partial ligamentous tears.

Throwers may have a structurally normal or abnormal MCL and may be pain-free or have pain with variable degrees of disability. These two factors (MCL integrity and pain) do not correlate precisely. Therefore, the critical issue in the throwing athlete is to determine whether the pain is arising from the MCL. To establish this diagnosis clearly, the history and physical examination must be considered.

The patient history should include at what point in the throwing motion the athlete experiences pain. Pain arising from the MCL is experienced at the point of maximum valgus torque in the elbow (ie, during the late cocking and early acceleration phases of throwing). For instance, medial elbow pain occurring principally during the follow-through phase is not from the MCL. On physical examination, an athlete with pain arising from the MCL due to valgus extension overload will have a positive moving valgus stress test[33] (**Figure 1**, *A*). This test was designed to reproduce the stresses on the elbow during the throwing motion. The shoulder is abducted 90°, and the elbow is maximally flexed. With the examiner supporting the humerus, a modest valgus torque is applied to the elbow until the shoulder reaches its limit of external rotation. While maintaining a constant valgus torque, the elbow is quickly extended to about 30°. Caution is required in patients with shoulder symptoms, which may be aggravated by this test. For an examination to be called positive, it must have two key components. First, the pain generated by the maneuver must reproduce the medial elbow pain at the MCL that the patient has with activities. Second, although the patient may experience pain throughout a range, the pain

FIGURE 1

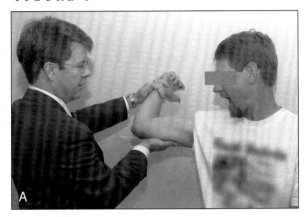
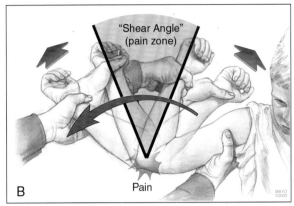

Moving valgus stress test. **A,** Starting with the arm in full flexion, the examiner applies a constant valgus torque to the elbow and then quickly extends the elbow. The patient experiences reproduction of his painful symptoms with an apprehension-like response in an arc as the elbow passes from 120° flexion to 70° of extension. **B,** Schematic representation of the moving valgus stress test. The shear range refers to the range of motion that causes pain while the elbow is being extended with valgus stress. The shear angle is the point that causes maximum pain. (Reproduced with permission from the Mayo Foundation, Rochester, MN.)

should be maximal between the position of late cocking and early acceleration (120° to 70°) as the elbow is extended. This specific angle of maximum pain is referred to as the "shear angle" (**Figure 1,** *B*). This examination technique has been shown to be highly sensitive (100%) and specific (75%).

I believe that the moving valgus stress test is sensitive because it recreates the actual stresses involved in the throwing motion. The same is true for other overhead sports such as tennis serves. Maximum valgus force in the throwing elbow has been demonstrated to occur between 120° and 90° of elbow flexion, the position the elbow is in during the acceleration phase. The greatest flexion angle occurs during the late cocking phase, and the elbow gradually extends during acceleration through release with flexion ranging from 98° during the cocking phase to 84° when the front foot contacts the ground to 23° at ball release[34,35] (**Figure 2**). Other authors have described the position of maximal elbow flexion to be 81° to 120°, occurring during the cocking phase.[35-38] The moment of maximal external rotation, or valgus load, is at approximately 65° of elbow flexion, and the most dramatic change in valgus loads occurs between 70° and 85° of elbow flexion.[38,39] As the elbow extends from the phase of front foot contact to release, compressive forces across the elbow increase. The contribution of bony articulation to elbow stability also increases, thus relieving the MCL of some of the valgus load through the

release phase.[40-43] These biomechanical principles are consistent with the data presented showing that patients with elbow MCL insufficiency experience pain with the moving valgus stress test during this late cocking (120°) to early acceleration (70°) phase.

I believe that injury to the MCL is a continuum, with three broad stages defined by the status of the collagen fibers and interfiber bonds of the anterior bundle of the MCL (**Figure 3**). In an elbow with stage 1 injury (debonding), valgus stress testing demonstrates no laxity (medial ulnohumeral joint opening). The exception would be a patient in whom prior asymptomatic attenuation of the ligament had led to laxity. In either case, surgical exploration would reveal no evidence of tearing of the ligament. In stage 2 (partial tear), some of the debonded collagen fibers tear. Healing with scar then usually occurs with the ligament in a lengthened, attenuated position. This results in functional lengthening of the ligament with evidence of laxity on valgus stress testing with radiographs and arthroscopy. In stage 3 (complete tear), the MCL ruptures completely, either as a result of having progressed through stages 1 and 2 (with or without symptoms), or from a sudden load that exceeded the strength of the ligament.

Establishing a diagnosis of elbow MCL insufficiency in an overhead athlete poses a significant challenge to the clinician and is usually based on a preponderance of the evidence (history, stress examination, and diag-

FIGURE 2

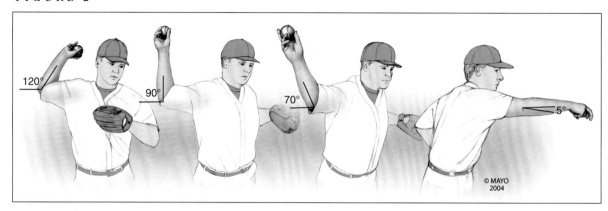

Pitching. As the elbow progresses through the acceleration phase, the elbow goes from a higher flexion angle to extension at ball release. Valgus torque at the elbow is increased throughout this phase from 120° to 70° of extension. (Reproduced with permission from the Mayo Foundation, Rochester, MN.)

FIGURE 3

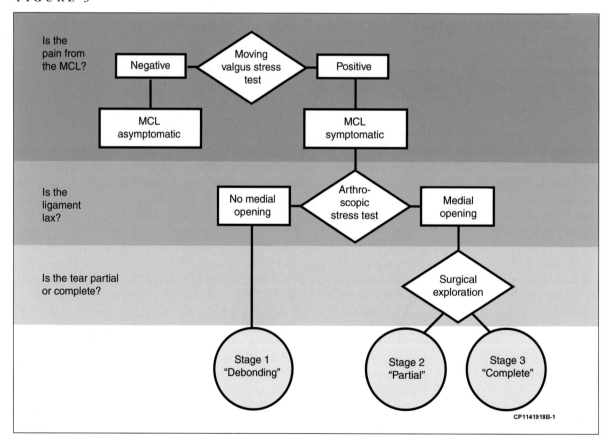

Algorithm using the moving valgus stress test to determine if the MCL is symptomatic. (Adapted with permission from the Mayo Foundation, Rochester, MN.)

nostic imaging). Frank Jobe, MD is a recognized authority on this topic and has contributed more to the understanding of the diagnosis and management of this injury than perhaps any other individual, and he and his colleagues still emphasize that the diagnosis rests on the patient history and physical examination.[14,15]

MRI can be confusing, and arthroscopic stress testing reveals more about laxity of the MCL than whether it may be a source of pain. A negative MRI or arthroscopic stress test does not effectively rule out insufficiency of the MCL. The moving valgus stress test gives insight into the dynamic forces that are occurring in the patient's elbow and is the most sensitive and specific tool in the diagnosis of symptomatic MCL insufficiency in throwing athletes. It has become common practice to perform MCL reconstruction if return to high-level throwing is desired and nonsurgical measures have failed, even in the absence of demonstrable laxity of the ligament by stress testing. However, it is critical to emphasize that this should be considered only if clinical examination confirms symptoms from the MCL with a positive moving valgus stress test. Such a patient would be considered to have a chronic stage 1 (debonding) MCL injury. On the other hand, in my practice I consider a normal moving valgus stress test to be a contraindication to MCL reconstruction. It is not unusual for me to accept a referral for an MCL reconstruction, only to find that the patient instead has one of the different conditions discussed below and can be returned to full participation in overhead sports without ever needing an MCL reconstruction.

The method of reconstruction has evolved somewhat since Jobe's original description. The advantages and disadvantages of different techniques relate to exposure, management of the ulnar nerve, and use of tunnels versus docking or screw interference techniques for securing the graft. Success rates have been high in returning athletes to their prior level of overhead sport.[44]

MEDIAL COMMON FLEXOR-PRONATOR TENDINITIS

The flexor-pronator musculature potentially stabilizes the elbow against valgus, but its role in MCL-deficient throwers is unclear. Flexor-pronator electromyographic activity is normally high in the late cocking and acceleration phases, ranging from 80% to 120% of maximum voluntary contraction, but MCL-deficient pitchers have been noted to exhibit decreased wrist flexor activity and increased wrist extensor activity.[8,45] Whether this is cause or effect is unknown. Clinically, muscular training is recommended for prevention and as part of nonsurgical and postoperative treatment.

Tendinitis of the common flexor-pronator tendons is probably much more common in throwers with medial elbow pain than recognized. Careful study of the anatomy of the tendon along with the anatomy of the underlying MCL reveals that a significant portion of the tendon can be thought of structurally as an augmentation of the underlying ligament itself. The tendon, which takes origin on the epicondyle, is structurally bonded to the ligament until it inserts on the ulna. Thus, the tendon origin experiences stress during throwing due to the dynamic muscle contraction of the common flexor-pronator group and the passively exerted valgus stresses transferred to the tendon due to its attachments on either side of the joint.

Diagnosis of medial common flexor-pronator tendinitis (medial epicondylitis, golfer's elbow, medial tennis elbow) can be challenging because of its frequent association with the other pain generators of the medial elbow, and the incidence in throwers is not known. Although the cause of the pain is debated, pathology specimens have demonstrated mucinous tendon degeneration within the muscle tendon fiber insertions. Anatomically, the fibers of the common flexor-pronator tendons and MCL are intermingled and lie adjacent to each other just distal to the origins, making diagnosis difficult.

Physical examination of patients with medial common flexor tendinitis demonstrates tenderness to palpation at the common flexor origin (specifically at the anterior aspect of the medial epicondyle with the elbow flexed to 90°) and pain with resisted pronation and/or flexion of the wrist. Common flexor tendinitis can be distinguished from symptomatic MCL pathology with the use of the moving valgus stress test (described above) and a medial tennis elbow shear test. My colleagues and I have substantial experience with the tennis elbow shear test for medial or lateral epicondylitis. The same principles of internal shear stresses used with the moving valgus stress test can be applied to this examination technique. With the elbow in the flexed position, the patient flexes and pronates the clenched fist against resistance applied by the examiner. The patient is then instructed to quickly extend the elbow. In the patient with medial tennis elbow syndrome, this maneuver will elicit the medial elbow pain that the patient is experiencing due to the internal shear forces within the tendon at the common flexor-pronator origin. I believe this test to be highly sensitive and specific. In my experience, approximately 24% of patients undergoing MCL reconstruction have clear and unequivocal evidence of medial epicondylitis in addition to MCL insufficiency requiring surgical treatment.

ULNAR NEURITIS AND NEUROPATHY

The ulnar nerve passes from the medial anterior compartment to the posterior compartment of the arm, passing through a thick intermuscular septum 8 to 10 cm proximal to the medial humeral epicondyle. The nerve passes posterior to the epicondyle and enters the cubital tunnel, which is defined by the medial trochlea, medial epicondylar groove, MCL complex, and the cubital tunnel retinaculum (roof). The ulnar nerve continues distally between the two heads of the flexor carpi ulnaris.

Ulnar nerve irritation or ulnar neuritis in athletes can be a source of debilitating medial elbow pain in throwers, and it may occur alone or in association with other clinical entities.[46] Ulnar nerve symptoms may manifest as localized medial elbow pain with paresthesias in the little and ring fingers that occur during the throwing motion. Players with ulnar nerve subluxation may also report a snapping sensation. More severe involvement (neuropathy) may manifest with pain at rest, diminished sensation in the ring and little fingers with progressive functional loss as indicated by loss of grip strength, and hand interossei atrophy.

In the absence of ulnar nerve subluxation, ulnar nerve irritation may be caused in part by reactive factors that occur about the elbow from repetitive use, resulting in abnormal compressive and traction forces on the ulnar nerve.[47] Medial elbow osteophytes may narrow the cubital tunnel with compression of the ulnar nerve.[48] Furthermore, the normal ulnar nerve gliding that occurs with flexion and extension may be inhibited by these points of impingement, further impairing nerve function.

Ulnar nerve irritation can be associated with medial elbow ligamentous insufficiency, which allows the elbow to open medially with the valgus torque of throwing and is thought to result in increased traction on the ulnar nerve with resultant symptoms. Ulnar nerve irritation can also occur due to friction in association with ulnar nerve subluxation or dislocation;[49] this happens as the ulnar nerve slides over the medial epicondyle with elbow flexion. Finally, local inflammation in the tendon or ligament may cause ulnar neuritis.

Physical examination of the medial elbow should include palpation of the ulnar nerve as it exits beneath the medial border of the triceps and approaches the medial humeral epicondyle. Gentle palpation can elicit exquisite pain with shock-like paresthesias to the ring and little fingers. Dynamic palpation of the ulnar nerve with elbow flexion and extension should also be performed to assess for medial subluxation of the ulnar nerve onto or over the medial epicondyle, which should normally be the most medial palpable structure. Subluxation may be partial or complete and can be associated with triceps subluxation. Neurologic examination includes bilateral sensory (with moving two-point testing) and motor examination (grip strength, pinch strength) to help assess the extent of neurologic deficit. Patients with more definite neurologic loss should undergo peripheral nerve studies preoperatively to clarify the extent of the loss. Electromyography can be useful; however, symptoms in most of these patients are transient, occurring only in the dynamic situation in which valgus stress is placed on the medial ulnohumeral joint. In such cases, stabilizing the elbow often is sufficient to manage the nerve symptoms.

MEDIAL TRICEPS TENDINITIS AND SNAPPING

Medial elbow pain associated with a snapping sensation is likely due to a subluxating-dislocating medial head of the triceps and is frequently associated with ulnar nerve subluxation and irritation. However, some of these patients are not aware of an actual snapping sensation. Triceps hypertrophy, which is commonly seen in throwing athletes or athletes who train with weights, is a risk factor for subluxating medial triceps, which typically occurs at flexion angles >90°.

Physical examination usually demonstrates above-average muscle mass and tenderness to palpation along the medial triceps muscle. If the medial epicondyle is firmly palpated while flexing the elbow from the extended position, first the ulnar nerve and then the

FIGURE 4

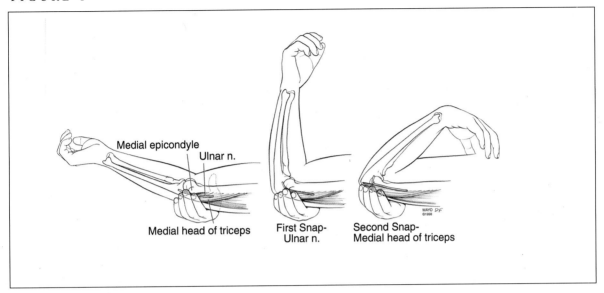

Examination of the medial elbow for subluxation of the ulnar nerve and medial triceps. With the examiner's finger placed over the medial epicondyle, active or passive elbow flexion demonstrates subluxation of the ulnar nerve as it passes over the edge of the medial epicondyle. If the triceps also subluxates, a second structure will be felt to pass over the medial epicondyle, often with a snap. Although ulnar nerve subluxation may exist in isolation, medial triceps subluxation is always associated with a subluxating ulnar nerve. (Reproduced with permission from the Mayo Foundation, Rochester, MN.)

medial triceps can be felt to subluxate around the epicondyle under the examiner's thumb (**Figure 4**). In fact, even if one presses very firmly, it is impossible to prevent the ulnar nerve and medial triceps from subluxating, and the more firmly they snap. Subluxation of the medial triceps onto or over the medial epicondyle can be elicited by resisted extension of the fully flexed elbow.[50] In my experience, extension against resistance may yield a palpable snap, usually before the elbow extends past 90°. Subluxation of the medial triceps is always associated with ulnar nerve dislocation or subluxation, and examination for both entities should be performed when one or the other is suspected.

Although snapping of the medial triceps is only rarely reported, this is likely due to a failure of proper diagnosis and has been frequently reported to be the cause of failed ulnar nerve transposition.[51] Failure to diagnose a snapping medial triceps in association with elbow MCL injury can also be a reason for continued medial elbow pain after an apparently successful ligament reconstruction. In my experience, 47% of patients undergoing MCL reconstruction have symptomatic medial triceps subluxation requiring treatment.

POSTEROMEDIAL IMPINGEMENT

Posteromedial impingement pain is a classic symptom in overhead athletes having valgus extension overload. It is worth noting, however, that the same problem is seen in patients with hypertrophic osteoarthritis of the elbow secondary to other causes. The patient reports sharp posterior or posteromedial pain at the end point of extension (ie, at ball release or follow-through). In most patients, an associated contracture of varying degrees is present.

In my practice, I have found that the diagnosis can be confirmed with confidence on physical examination using the following provocative tests: the extension impingement test and the arm bar test. The extension impingement test is performed by starting with the elbow near full extension, then quickly (but gently, so as to not injure the patient) snapping it into terminal extension. This maneuver reproduces the posterior or posteromedial pain experienced during throwing. Simultaneous valgus load will normally enhance the pain, which will usually diminish with a varus load.

FIGURE 5

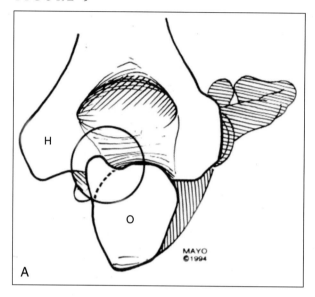 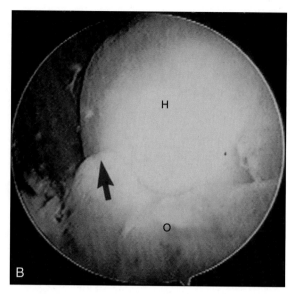

Drawing **(A)** and arthroscopic view **(B)** demonstrating osteophytes (arrow) on the posteromedial olecranon. Such osteophytes, which are common in overhead throwing athletes due to valgus extension overload, can limit extension but do not necessarily cause pain unless they have fractured and progressed to a nonunion. H = humerus, O = olecranon. (Part A reproduced with permission from the Mayo Foundation, Rochester, MN.)

Another similar test is the arm bar test, which is a variation of a martial arts maneuver. With the patient's shoulder in 90° of forward elevation and full internal rotation and the patient's hand placed on the shoulder of the examiner, the examiner then pulls down on the olecranon, leveraging the elbow into extension. Again, reproduction of the patient's pain due to impingement is expected if such pathology is present. I have found this test to be perhaps more sensitive if the patient's symptoms are relatively minor or have diminished just before consultation.

Although the patient may have osteophytes on the posteromedial olecranon, osteophytes alone do not always cause impingement pain (**Figure 5**). In fact, the relationship between bony osteophytes and impingement pain poses an apparent dilemma. It is not unusual to see osteophytes that impinge at the limit of motion in patients who have no pain. Therefore, the question is why some osteophytes are painful and others are not. Based on experience and unpublished research in progress, I believe that the usual cause for impingement pain in such circumstances is a fractured olecranon osteophyte that has typically progressed to nonunion by the time of referral to the orthopaedic surgeon. Such fracture-nonunions are best visualized on CT scans with sagittal and coronal reconstructions (**Figure 6**). The loose fragment is easily missed during arthroscopy because it is either very small or covered with cartilage and not obviously "loose." In some patients, the loose fragment is removed during osteophyte excision without ever being recognized. Other causes for the pain can include loose bodies or buildup of inflamed soft tissue posteriorly.

Patient history can provide so much evidence of a (nonunited) fractured olecranon osteophyte that it has become what I refer to as a "telephone diagnosis." In a baseball pitcher or catcher, the pain is felt posteriorly or posteromedially at terminal extension, at or after ball release. It does not cause pain in the cocking or acceleration phases of throwing because there is no actual impingement until the elbow is fully extended. A positive extension impingement test or arm bar test is highly sensitive (and relatively highly specific) for posteromedial impingement caused by a nonunited fractured olecranon osteophyte. A patient who has other causes of pain, such as an MCL injury, will be able to distinguish two separate types of pain if asked specifically.

The best imaging study is CT with two-dimensional

FIGURE 6

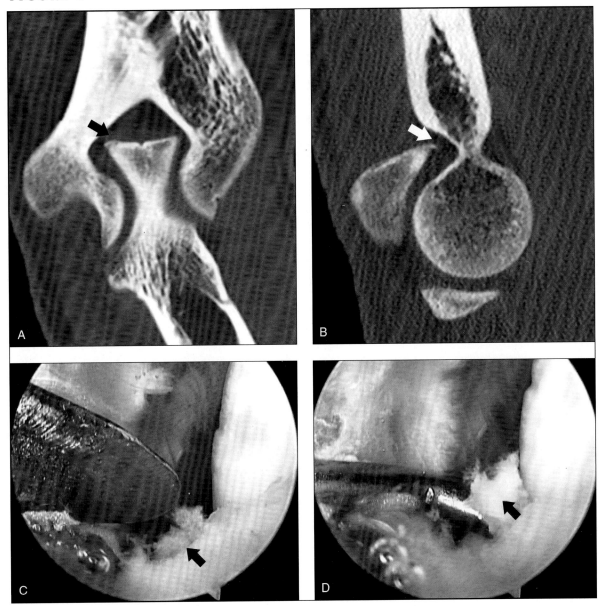

Posteromedial impingement due to a nonunited fracture of an olecranon osteophyte in a 20-year-old college pitcher seen for undiagnosed persistent posteromedial elbow pain for two seasons. Sagittal **(A)** and coronal **(B)** CT reconstructions show a tiny nonunited fractured osteophyte at the posteromedial corner of the olecranon (arrows). C and D are arthroscopic views of the posteromedial olecranon. In **C,** the posteromedial corner of the olecranon is being explored with a periosteal elevator and a cleavage line is identified between the tiny osteophyte that is nonunited to the rest of the olecranon (arrow). In **D,** the nonunion fragment (arrow) is being lifted away from the olecranon with a blunt probe. After simple excision of this fragment and removal of soft tissue from the olecranon fossa, this patient experienced complete relief of pain and at 6 weeks postoperatively had returned to full pitching without pain or limitation. His extension impingement test and arm bar test, which had both been positive preoperatively, were negative 6 weeks postoperatively.

FIGURE 7

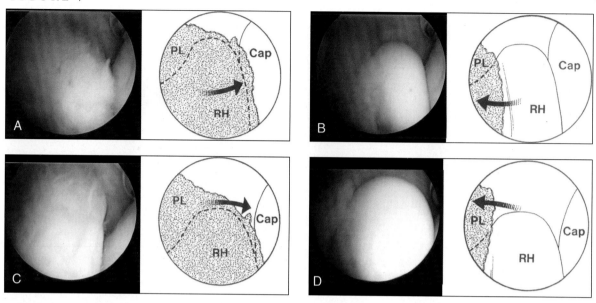

Arthroscopic and corresponding schematic views of the plica falling into the radiohumeral articulation with extension (**A** and **C**) and retracting with flexion (**B** and **D**). PL = plica, RH = radial head, Cap = capitellum. (Adapted with permission from Antuna SA, O'Driscoll SW: Snapping plicae associated with radiocapitellar chondromalacia. *Arthroscopy* 2001;17:491-495.)

FIGURE 8

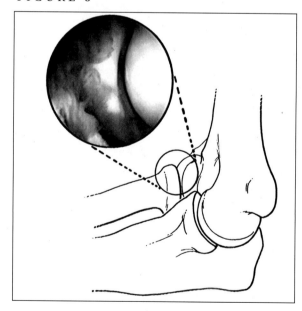

Arthroscopic view shows a localized area of synovitis around the radial head. This is a common finding when first entering the joint. (Reproduced with permission from Antuna SA, O'Driscoll SW: Snapping plicae associated with radiocapitellar chondromalacia. *Arthroscopy* 2001;17:491-495.)

sagittal and coronal reconstructions and three-dimensional surface rendering to show the overall morphologic changes.

The indication for surgical treatment of posteromedial impingement is clinical and is predicated on confirmation that the patient's symptoms are caused by the impingement with a positive extension impingement test and/or arm bar test. In fact, I believe that posteromedial decompression is contraindicated if neither of these tests is positive, regardless of pathologic changes seen on imaging studies or at the time of surgery.

Treatment of symptomatic posteromedial impingement includes removal of any nonunited fractured osteophyte and the pathologic bone (osteophyte), not just from the posterior and posteromedial olecranon, but also from the olecranon fossa and from between the posteromedial trochlea and medial epicondyle. No normal bone should be removed from the olecranon as this would shorten the moment arm, providing a fulcrum against which valgus torque is resisted by the MCL. Shortening the olecranon increases strain in the MCL, placing it at risk of subsequent failure.[52,53] If any doubt remains regarding adequacy of decompression, additional bone removal should be performed on the humeral side, not the olecranon. This operation is typically performed arthroscopically, so a word of caution is appropriate. The ulnar nerve is at risk of being wound up and injured by a spinning burr, so appropriate measures should be taken to avoid this.

CHONDRAL EROSION ON THE POSTEROMEDIAL TROCHLEA

Chondral erosions on the posteromedial trochlea can occur as a result of chronic valgus overload. They typically cause pain in the deceleration phase of throwing. Although they are not common, they can be suspected based on the history (timing of pain) and the presence of a positive chondral shear test. This test is basically a moving valgus stress test, but instead of pain being present between 70° and 120°, it is present in extension (short of terminal extension). Optimum treatment has not been determined, but microfracture has been satisfactory in my experience.

SNAPPING PLICA

The presence of synovial plicae is a well-recognized cause of clinical symptoms in the knee joint.[54] These structures become inflamed and thickened, sometimes due to trauma, and impinge or snap in the joint. A similar condition is described in the elbow.

Ogilvie[55] and Trethowan[56] described the presence of a synovial fringe at the periphery of the radiocapitellar joint. They believed that it could be compressed between the radial head and humerus, causing inflammation and pain. Caputo and associates[57] described it as a meniscus-like fibrocartilage similar to the knee meniscus and found abundant nerve endings in its periphery, inferring the possibility of pain directly associated with pathology in this structure. They inferred from their observation that a painful plica may mimic lateral epicondylitis and that the pain from such a condition would be relieved by excision of the inflamed plica. Other authors have suggested excision of this synovial fringe as part of the surgical treatment of tennis elbow.[58-60]

Clarke[61] and Antuna and O'Driscoll[62] documented an association between chondromalacia on the margin of the radial head and snapping plica. In a report of 14 patients, 9 had a history of trauma[62] (**Figure 7**). It is possible that even after minor trauma, a synovial reaction

can produce inflammation of this synovial fold that with time becomes enlarged and thickened (**Figure 8**). Repetitive movements of the joint, especially in extension and pronation, can perpetuate the irritation and produce chronic localized synovitis. Abrasion is most likely responsible for the chondromalacia seen on the radial head over which the plica snaps.

Pain localized in the lateral aspect of the elbow and the reproduction of symptoms during flexion-extension of the pronated forearm should lead the physician to consider the possibility of a synovial plica in the radiocapitellar joint. Antuna and O'Driscoll[62] reported the plica impingement test to be a diagnostic physical examination maneuver for radiocapitellar plicae. The plica impingement test involves loading the elbow into valgus and then passively flexing it to the limit of flexion while holding the forearm pronated (flexion-pronation test) for an anterior plica. A posterior plica is diagnosed with the extension-supination plica impingement test, by extending the elbow to its limit while holding it in supination and valgus. Gentle thumb pressure over the posterior radiocapitellar joint assists with obtaining a painful snap. For both tests, a painful snap at the radiocapitellar joint is a positive test. When the diagnosis is suspected, arthroscopy has proved to be useful both as a diagnostic and therapeutic tool.

For three reasons, the diagnosis may be missed clinically. First, with so little literature and teaching devoted to the topic of plicae in the elbow, the phenomenon does not rank high on the list of differential diagnoses. Second, the clinical examination and list of differential diagnoses for snapping at the elbow are not familiar to many clinicians. Third, the lateral location of the pain, and the typical tenderness over the radiocapitellar region, make a misdiagnosis of tennis elbow likely. This is particularly likely if the clinician focuses more on the symptom of pain than the symptom of snapping.

Arthroscopic excision of the plica typically results in complete resolution of the snapping. Care must be taken not to damage the annular ligament or the articular surfaces of the radial head and capitellum.

REFERENCES

1. Bennett G: Shoulder and elbow lesions of the professional baseball pitcher. *JAMA* 1941;117:510-514.
2. Waris W: Elbow injuries of javelin throwers. *Acta Chir Scand* 1946;93:563-575.

3. Slocum DB: Classification of elbow injuries from baseball pitching. *Tex Med* 1968;64:48-53.

4. King J, Brelsford HJ, Tullos HS: Analysis of the pitching arm of the professional baseball pitcher. *Clin Orthop Relat Res* 1969;67:116-123.

5. Sakurai S, Ikegami Y, Okamoto A, Yabe K, Toyoshima S: A three-dimensional cinematographic analysis of upper limb movement during the fastball and curveball baseball pitches. *J Appl Biomech* 1993;9:47-65.

6. Giangarra CE, Conroy B, Jobe FW, Pink M, Perry J: Electromyographic and cinematographic analysis of elbow function in tennis players using single- and double-handed backhand strokes. *Am J Sports Med* 1993;21:394-399.

7. DiGiovine NM, Jobe FW, Pink M, Perry J: An electromyographic analysis of the upper extremity in pitching. *J Shoulder Elbow Surg* 1992;1:15-25.

8. Hamilton CD, Glousman RE, Jobe FW, Brault J, Pink M, Perry J: Dynamic stability of the elbow: Electromyographic analysis of the flexor pronator group and the extensor group in pitchers with valgus instability. *J Shoulder Elbow Surg* 1996;5:347-354.

9. Fleisig GS, Barrentine SW, Escamilla RF, Andrews JR: Biomechanics of overhand throwing with implications for injuries. *Sports Med* 1996;21:421-437.

10. Peterson RK, Savoie FH III, Field LD: Osteochondritis dissecans of the elbow. *Instr Course Lect* 1999;48:393-398.

11. Brooks AA: Stress fractures of the upper extremity. *Clin Sports Med* 2001;20:613-620.

12. Cain EL Jr, Dugas JR, Wolf RS, Andrews JR: Elbow injuries in throwing athletes: A current concepts review. *Am J Sports Med* 2003;31:621-635.

13. Conway JE, Jobe FW, Glousman RE, Pink M: Medial instability of the elbow in throwing athletes. *J Bone Joint Surg Am* 1992;74:67-83.

14. Jobe F, ElAttrache N: Diagnosis and treatment of ulnar collateral ligament injuries in athletes, in Morrey B (ed): *The Elbow and Its Disorders*, ed 3. Philadelphia, PA, WB Saunders Co, 2000, pp 549-555.

15. Jobe FW, Stark H, Lombardo S: Reconstruction of the ulnar collateral ligament in athletes. *J Bone Joint Surg Am* 1986;68:1158-1163.

16. Kuroda S, Sakamaki K: Ulnar collateral ligament tears of the elbow joint. *Clin Orthop Relat Res* 1986;208:266-271.

17. Safran MR: Elbow injuries in athletes. *Clin Orthop Relat Res* 1995;310:257-277.

18. Bennett J, Mehlhoff T: Articular injuries in the athlete, in Morrey B (ed): *The Elbow and its Disorders*, ed 3. Philadelphia, PA, WB Saunders Co, 2000, pp 563-575.

19. Wilson FD, Andrews JR, Blackburn TA, McCluskey G: Valgus extension overload in the pitching elbow. *Am J Sports Med* 1983;11:83-88.

20. Andrews JR, Wilk KE, Satterwhite YE, Tedder JL: Physical examination of the thrower's elbow. *J Orthop Sports Phys Ther* 1993;17:296-304.

21. Callaway GH, Field LD, Deng XH, et al: Biomechanical evaluation of the medial collateral ligament of the elbow. *J Bone Joint Surg Am* 1997;79:1223-1231.

22. Lee GA, Katz SD, Lazarus MD: Elbow valgus stress radiography in an uninjured population. *Am J Sports Med* 1998;26:425-427.

23. Rijke AM, Goitz HT, McCue FC, Andrews JR, Berr SS: Stress radiography of the medial elbow ligaments. *Radiology* 1994;191:213-216.

24. Ellenbecker TS, Mattalino AJ, Elam EA, Caplinger RA: Medial elbow joint laxity in professional baseball pitchers: A bilateral comparison using stress radiography. *Am J Sports Med* 1998;26:420-424.

25. De Smet AA, Winter TC, Best TM, Bernhardt DT: Dynamic sonography with valgus stress to assess elbow ulnar collateral ligament injury in baseball pitchers. *Skeletal Radiol* 2002;31:671-676.

26. Fritz RC, Steinbach LS: Magnetic resonance imaging of the musculoskeletal system: Part 3. The elbow. *Clin Orthop Relat Res* 1996;324:321-339.

27. Mirowitz SA, London SL: Ulnar collateral ligament injury in baseball pitchers: MR imaging evaluation. *Radiology* 1992;185:573-576.

28. Schwartz ML, al-Zahrani S, Morwessel RM, Andrews JR: Ulnar collateral ligament injury in the throwing athlete: Evaluation with saline-enhanced MR arthrography. *Radiology* 1995;197:297-299.

29. Timmerman LA, Schwartz ML, Andrews JR: Preoperative evaluation of the ulnar collateral ligament by magnetic resonance imaging and computed tomography arthrography: Evaluation in 25 baseball players with surgical confirmation. *Am J Sports Med* 1994;22:26-31.

30. Timmerman LA, Andrews JR: Histology and arthroscopic anatomy of the ulnar collateral ligament of the elbow. *Am J Sports Med* 1994;22:667-673.

31. Timmerman LA, Andrews JR: Undersurface tear of the ulnar collateral ligament in baseball players: A newly recognized lesion. *Am J Sports Med* 1994;22:33-36.

32. Field LD, Altchek DW: Evaluation of the arthroscopic valgus instability test of the elbow. *Am J Sports Med* 1996;24:177-181.

33. O'Driscoll SW, Lawton RL, Smith AM: The "moving valgus stress test" for medial collateral ligament tears of the elbow. *Am J Sports Med* 2005;33:231-239.

34. Fleisig GS, Barrentine SW, Zheng N, Escamilla RF, Andrews JR: Kinematic and kinetic comparison of baseball pitching among various levels of development. *J Biomech* 1999;32:1371-1375.

35. Fleisig GS, Escamilla RF, Andrews JR, Matsuo T, Satter-white Y, Barrentine SW: Kinematic and kinetic comparison between baseball pitching and football passing. *J Appl Biomech* 1996;12:207-224.

36. Feltner M, Dapena J: Dynamics of the shoulder and elbow joints of the throwing arm during a baseball pitch. *Int J Sports Biomech* 1986;2:235-259.

37. Pappas AM, Zawacki RM, Sullivan TJ: Biomechanics of baseball pitching: A preliminary report. *Am J Sports Med* 1985;13:216-222.

38. Werner SL, Fleisig GS, Dillman CJ, Andrews JR: Biomechanics of the elbow during baseball pitching. *J Orthop Sports Phys Ther* 1993;17:274-278.

39. Escamilla R, Fleisig G, Barrentine S, Zheng N, Andrews J: Kinematic comparisons of throwing different types of baseball pitches. *J Appl Biomech* 1998;14:1-23.

40. Hotchkiss RN, Weiland AJ: Valgus stability of the elbow. *J Orthop Res* 1987;5:372-377.

41. Morrey BF, An K-N, Tanaka S: Valgus stability of the elbow: A definition of primary and secondary constraints. *Clin Orthop Relat Res* 1991;265:187-195.

42. O'Driscoll SW: Elbow instability. *Hand Clin* 1994;10:405-415.

43. Sojbjerg JO, Ovesen J, Nielsen S: Experimental elbow instability after transection of the medial collateral ligament. *Clin Orthop Relat Res* 1987;218:186-190.

44. Dodson CC, Thomas A, Dines JS, Nho SJ, Williams RJ III, Altchek DW: Medial ulnar collateral ligament reconstruction of the elbow in throwing athletes. *Am J Sports Med* 2006;34:1926-1932.

45. Davidson PA, Pink M, Perry J, Jobe FW: Functional anatomy of the flexor pronator muscle group in relation to the medial collateral ligament of the elbow. *Am J Sports Med* 1995;23:245-250.

46. Glousman RE: Ulnar nerve problems in the athlete's elbow. *Clin Sports Med* 1990;9:365-377.

47. Del Pizzo W, Jobe FW, Norwood L: Ulnar nerve entrapment syndrome in baseball players. *Am J Sports Med* 1977;5:182-185.

48. O'Driscoll SW, Horii E, Morrey BF, Carmichael SW: The cubital tunnel and ulnar neuropathy. *J Bone Joint Surg Br* 1991;73:613-617.

49. Childress HM: Recurrent ulnar nerve dislocation at the elbow. *Clin Orthop Relat Res* 1975;108:168-173.

50. Spinner RJ, Goldner RD: Snapping of the medial head of the triceps and recurrent dislocation of the ulnar nerve. *J Bone Joint Surg Am* 1998;80:239-247.

51. Spinner RJ, O'Driscoll S, Jupiter J, Goldner R: Unrecognized dislocation of the medial portion of the triceps: Another cause of failed ulnar nerve transposition. *J Neurosurg* 2000;92:52-57.

52. Ahmad CS, Park MC, Elattrache NS: Elbow medial ulnar collateral ligament insufficiency alters posteromedial olecranon contact. *Am J Sports Med* 2004;32:1607-1612.

53. Kamineni S, ElAttrache NS, O'Driscoll SW, et al: Medial collateral ligament strain with partial posteromedial olecranon resection: A biomechanical study. *J Bone Joint Surg Am* 2004;86:2424-2430.

54. Jackson R, Patel D: Synovial lesions: Plicae, in McGinty J, Caspari R, Jackson R, Poehling G (eds): *Operative Arthroscopy*. New York, NY, Lippincott-Raven, 1996, pp 447-458.

55. Ogilvie W: Discussion on minor injuries of the elbow joint. *Proc R Soc Med* 1929;23:306-322.

56. Trethowan W: Tennis elbow. *BMJ* 1929;2:1218.

57. Caputo A, Hartford C, Proia A, Urbaniak J: The radiocapitellar meniscal complex: An anatomical and histological analysis. Proceedings of the 54th Annual Meeting of the American Society for Surgery of the Hand. Boston, MA, September 2-4, 1999 (paper 19).

58. Moore M Jr: Radiohumeral synovitis: A cause of persistent elbow pain. *Surg Clin North Am* 1953;Oct:1363-1371.

59. Nirschl RP, Pettrone FA: Tennis elbow: The surgical treatment of lateral epicondylitis. *J Bone Joint Surg Am* 1979;61:832-839.

60. Stack J, Hunt W: Radio-humeral synovitis. *Q Bull Northwest Univ Med School* 1946;20:394-397.

61. Clarke RP: Symptomatic, lateral synovial fringe (plica) of the elbow joint. *Arthroscopy* 1988;4:112-116.

62. Antuna SA, O'Driscoll SW: Snapping plicae associated with radiocapitellar chondromalacia. *Arthroscopy* 2001;17:491-495.

CHAPTER 8

ARTHROSCOPIC
OSTEOCAPSULAR ARTHROPLASTY

ROBERT Z. TASHJIAN, MD
KEN YAMAGUCHI, MD

Elbow arthritis is a relatively common cause of elbow pain and dysfunction; although not common in young athletes, it can become a problem later in life. Etiologies include trauma, rheumatoid arthritis, osteochondritis, and primary degenerative arthritis. Primary degenerative arthritis largely affects middle-aged men. Patients present with impingement pain at the extremes of motion and mild flexion and extension contractures.[1] Pain in the midrange of elbow motion is uncommon in the setting of early primary degenerative arthritis but is often present in posttraumatic and end-stage rheumatoid arthritis and osteoarthritis. The pathoanatomy of primary degenerative arthritis comprises olecranon and coronoid process osteophytes; bony overgrowth in the olecranon, radial head, and coronoid fossae; loose bodies; and marginal posteromedial and lateral gutter osteophytes. All of these ultimately cause pain and stiffness. The ulnohumeral and radiohumeral cartilage is relatively preserved. Débridement of excess bone and capsular release is a reasonable treatment alternative for patients who have impingement pain with early arthritis but do not have significant articular cartilage loss.

Surgical treatment options for symptomatic patients with elbow arthritis who have relatively preserved articular surfaces include open and arthroscopic débridement. Open débridement (the Outerbridge-Kashiwagi procedure) was originally described by Kashiwagi in 1978.[2] The Outerbridge-Kashiwagi procedure includes olecranon tip resection, transhumeral fenestration, and coronoid tip resection. Morrey modified the Outerbridge-Kashiwagi procedure and called it ulnohumeral arthroplasty.[3] He uses a trephine for fenestration, along with elevation of the triceps rather than splitting it to expose the olecranon.

Arthroscopic methods of débridement, including a modified ulnohumeral arthroplasty procedure (with and without humeral fenestration), also have been described.[4-7] Redden and Stanley[6] originally reported on arthroscopic posterior fenestration alone. This technique was later modified to include posterior compartment osteophyte débridement along with humeral fenestration.[5] Savoie and associates[7] further modified the Ogilvie-Harris technique[5] by adding an anterior and posterior capsular release, anterior bony débridement through anterior portals, and radial head resection. O'Driscoll[4] suggested that fenestration is not required but rather emphasized complete removal of excess osteophytic bone both anteriorly (coronoid and radial head fossa) and posteriorly (olecranon fossa, medial and lateral gutters), along with loose body removal and anterior/posterior capsular release.

Currently, arthroscopic osteocapsular arthroplasty is an effective treatment option for patients with moderate elbow arthritis as long as the surgeon has significant experience in performing elbow arthroscopy. The current technique of arthroscopic osteocapsular arthroplasty includes anterior bony débridement (radial head fossa, coronoid fossa, coronoid tip, possible radial head resection, anterolateral distal humeral osteophytes), anterior capsular release, posterior bony débridement (olecranon fossa with or without humeral fenestration, posteromedial and lateral gutters, olecranon tip), posterior capsular release, posterolateral plicae excision, and loose body removal. Clinical results following arthroscopic osteocapsular arthroplasty are promising at mid-term, with preserved gains in flexion arc and decreased pain levels comparable to results following open ulno-humeral arthroplasty. The indications, contraindications, technique, and results of arthroscopic osteocapsular arthroplasty are reviewed in this chapter.

INDICATIONS

The principal indication for arthroscopic osteocapsular arthroplasty is symptomatic primary degenerative osteoarthritis of the elbow with restricted motion and end–range-of-motion pain. Pain is commonly derived from excess bone at the olecranon and coronoid tips impinging on bone in their respective fossae. The goals of surgery are to improve motion and impingement pain. Relative indications include posttraumatic arthritis with preserved articular joint surfaces. Caution should be exercised in patients with significant posttraumatic deformity of the distal humerus and radial head because scarred capsule in the anterolateral aspect of the joint places the radial nerve at risk during débridement and capsular release. Hypertrophic inflammatory arthritis may also be treated with osteocapsular arthroplasty including synovectomy. These patients routinely have more advanced involvement of the articular cartilage, however, which limits the value of the procedure in this patient population.

CONTRAINDICATIONS

Disease severity dictates treatment in patients with elbow arthritis. Osteocapsular arthroplasty is primarily indicated for patients with mild to moderate arthritis. When midrange motion pain exists with severe bone loss, articular damage, or deformity, total elbow arthroplasty or interposition arthroplasty is a better surgical treatment option with more predictable long-term results.

To perform elbow arthroscopy safely, an extensive knowledge of elbow bony and neurovascular anatomy is required. For advanced procedures such as osteocapsular arthroplasty, in which neurovascular injury is a significant risk, extensive experience with elbow arthroscopy is mandatory. Therefore, surgeon unfamiliarity with elbow arthroscopy is a contraindication for this procedure.

The ulnar nerve is at significant risk during the development of medial portals, especially if the patient has had prior ulnar nerve surgery. Also, anterior capsular release is hazardous when the ulnar nerve has been mobilized in a submuscular sling. Therefore, an absolute contraindication for arthroscopic osteocapsular arthroplasty is a prior submuscular ulnar nerve transposition. If a prior subcutaneous nerve transposition has been performed, avoidance of anterior medial portal placement is strongly advised unless the ulnar nerve can be identified and protected. Posterior compartment arthroscopy can be safely performed in the setting of prior transposition and may be used to augment an open débridement of the anterior compartment.

Finally, several open procedures may be required in the surgical treatment of arthritis, including hardware removal, ulnar nerve transposition, or ligament reconstruction. It may be more prudent to perform an open débridement and release when combining osteocapsular arthroplasty with other procedures that require extensive surgical dissection.

TECHNIQUE

Initial Setup

Arthroscopic osteocapsular arthroplasty of the elbow is one of the more technically difficult procedures to perform. Proper setup and portal placement is essential to achieving a good outcome. We prefer general anesthesia. The patient is placed in the lateral decubitus position, which is better suited to this procedure than the supine position because much of the procedure is performed in the posterior compartment of the elbow. The lateral decubitus position allows ready access to the posterior compartment with a stable arm that can be easily extended (**Figure 1**).

Standard equipment includes a 4.5-mm, 30° large-joint arthroscope. Small-joint arthroscopes are not usually necessary. A special low-flow sheath without periarticular perforations should be used to minimize subcutaneous fluid extravasation. Only blunt trochars are used, and a pump is routinely used with the pressure set to as low a setting as possible to provide visualization. A tourniquet is always used, so high-pressure flow is not necessary to obtain hemostasis. Cannulas are generally not necessary and are usually avoided to allow free mobility of the instruments.

Additional equipment includes a multipolar cautery device for rapid tissue ablation, blunt switching sticks to place portals, and narrow-lane elevators to provide retraction. Specialized retractors are also available if necessary. Finally, we prefer to use guidewires and cannulated expanders to localize and establish correct portal locations.

Arthroscopic Portals

A multitude of portals have been described for elbow arthroscopy.[8] The basic portals generally used for arthroscopic osteocapsular arthroplasty include an anterolateral portal and an anteromedial portal for work in the anterior elbow. Posterior portals include a posterolateral and posterior portal. Finally, a midlateral portal is used. Accessory portals can also be used for retractors as necessary.

Retractors offer the advantages that soft tissues, including neurovascular structures, can be safely elevated away from sharp instrumentation and visualization can be maintained without significant fluid distention. The disadvantages of retractors include the necessity of skilled assistance, increased number of portals, and "crowding" of a small articular space.

Surgical Goals

Arthroscopic elbow osteocapsular arthroplasty involves both the soft tissues and the bony anatomy. Generally, soft-tissue contraction of both the posterior and anterior capsules is present to some extent, so releases of these capsules are usually necessary. When elbow flexion is limited to less than 100° to 110°, a specific release of the posterior bundle of the medial collateral ligament is also necessary.

Specific areas of bony débridement are generally targeted with arthroscopic osteocapsular arthroplasty. In the anterior compartment of the elbow, these include (1) humeral osteophytes in the radial head fossa proximal to the capitellum; (2) humeral osteophytes in the coronoid fossa proximal to the trochlear articular cartilage; (3) coronoid tip osteophytes; and (4) loose bodies, and occasionally osteophytes, from the coronoid on the anterior side of the lesser sigmoid notch. In the posterior compartment, targets of bony débridement include (1) olecranon fossa osteophytes, generally seen as a ridge extending across the fossa along its medial to lateral width; (2) olecranon tip osteophytes, which must be removed all along its medial to lateral extent; (3) posterior capitellar osteophytes just posterior to the articular surface; and (4) loose bodies.

FIGURE 1

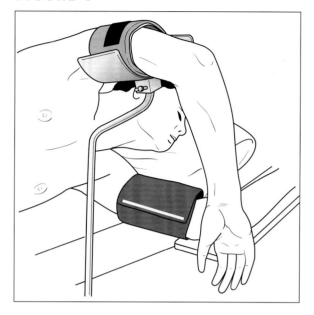

Patient in lateral decubitus position with arm in arm holder and nonsterile tourniquet applied. (Reproduced from Yamaguchi K, Tashjian RZ: Setup and portals, in Yamaguchi K, King GJW, McKee MD, O'Driscoll SW (eds): *Advanced Reconstruction Elbow.* Rosemont, IL, American Academy of Orthopaedic Surgeons, 2007, p 5.)

Procedure

Controversy exists regarding which compartment of the elbow is best for initiation of the procedure. We prefer starting with the anterior compartment because of concerns for radial nerve injury. The radial nerve is the nerve most at risk with elbow arthroscopy, and performing anterior arthroscopy first provides the advantage of performing this procedure before significant fluid distention and thus increased danger to the radial nerve. Others prefer starting in the posterior compartment because this portion of the procedure can be the most challenging in terms of bony work.

For anterior compartment arthroscopy, anterolateral and anteromedial portals are preferred to the alternative proximal anterolateral and proximal anteromedial portals. Although the proximal portals allow a greater safety margin to the overlying radial and median nerves, they restrict angle access to débride important osteophytes in the anterior compartment (**Figure 2**). Thus, the portals preferred for this procedure are closer to nerves. Care should be taken to obtain the necessary experience to perform this

FIGURE 2

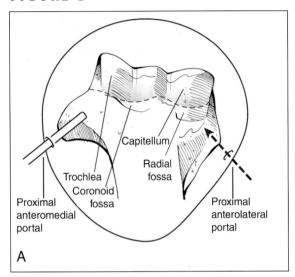
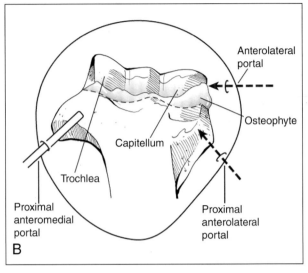

Drawings illustrating the advantage of the anterolateral portal when osteophytes are present. **A,** Axial view of the distal humerus as seen with the camera in the proximal anteromedial portal. The arrow indicates the direction of entry for the proximal anterolateral portal. **B,** Axial view of the distal humerus in an osteoarthritic elbow. The anterolateral portal (top arrow) is required instead of the proximal anterolateral portal (bottom arrow) to gain entry past lateral osteophytes. (Reproduced from Yamaguchi K, Tashjian RZ: Setup and portals, in Yamaguchi K, King GJW, McKee MD, O'Driscoll SW (eds): *Advanced Reconstruction Elbow*. Rosemont, IL, American Academy of Orthopaedic Surgeons, 2007, p 7.)

procedure safely when using the more dangerous portals.

We prefer to enter the elbow joint from the medial side first. It is important to enter the joint as medially as possible and not slide into the joint at a more central location. Once a medial portal is established, a lateral portal is then obtained under direct visualization. This ensures accurate portal placement in a safe location for this more dangerous anterolateral portal. A guidewire is placed percutaneously directly over the radiocapitellar joint (**Figure 3**). Once appropriate positioning of the guidewire is verified arthroscopically, an incision is made over the guidewire and the portal is dilated with cannulated switching sticks. If the joint is heavily contracted and the available visualization is limited, the guidewire is removed and the switching stick is used to bluntly elevate the contracted anterior capsule off the humerus in a sweeping motion (**Figure 4**). This offers a safe method to improve the joint space available for débridement.

A full-radius resector is generally inserted next, and a débridement of loose synovial tissue is performed to improve visualization of the joint space. Sweeping the capsule off the anterior humerus and performing a synovial débridement with a shaver usually provides sufficient joint space visualization for performing bony work. If this is

not the case, then a formal capsular release is performed. This is done under direct visualization from the medial side by placing a capsular biter through the lateral portal. Care must be taken to keep the biter directly on the capsule laterally, as the radial nerve is nearby. These initial bites on the lateral side should be performed with the biter directed in a proximal-medial direction to stay as far as possible from the radial nerve. Once a plane is established, further release of the capsule medially is generally safe because the brachialis muscle protects the overlying medial nerve and brachial artery from injury. A burr is then inserted laterally and osteophytes are removed. Radial head fossa osteophytes are removed first, followed by osteophytes just proximal to the lateral ridge of the trochlea. This improves visualization and access of instruments into the medial compartment. Generally, the burr is continued along from lateral toward medial all the way to the coronoid fossa, which can be accessed quite well if the anterolateral portal location is placed accurately. The arthroscope is redirected into the lateral portal using switching sticks, and the burr is then placed in the medial portal. Osteophytes remaining within the coronoid fossa are removed via this medial portal. Remaining coronoid tip osteophytes are then removed via this medial portal. Some flexion of

FIGURE 3

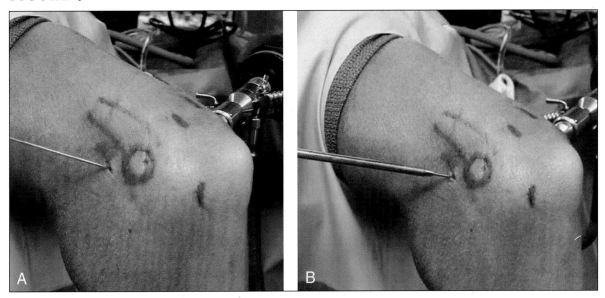

Procedure for portal placement. **A,** Guidewire localization of the proximal anterolateral portal. **B,** Portal tract expansion with cannulated dilators before cannula placement. (Reproduced from Yamaguchi K, Tashjian RZ: Setup and portals, in Yamaguchi K, King GJW, McKee MD, O'Driscoll SW (eds): *Advanced Reconstruction Elbow.* Rosemont, IL, American Academy of Orthopaedic Surgeons, 2007, p 4.)

the elbow is generally necessary to achieve full débridement of the coronoid tip. Generally, the burr is used to remove bony structures down to the coronoid articular cartilage. At this point, the remaining articular cartilage is easily removed using a biter or grasping tool. Use of the burr is avoided to prevent inadvertent entry to articular surfaces.

Posterior Compartment Arthroscopy

Posterior arthroscopy is started at the posterolateral portal. Generally the arthroscope is placed from the posterolateral portal directly into the olecranon fossa. Using a blunt trochar tip, a sweeping motion is made from distal to proximal, releasing the posterior capsule from the olecranon fossa and improving the space for visualization. After proper fluid distention posteriorly, a central posterior portal is then established under direct visualization. A full radius resector or multipolar electrocautery device is used to débride the posterior fat pad and synovial tissues to improve visualization. Sharp instruments such as a shaver are used with the back of the instrument facing medially, to minimize the risk of injuring the ulnar nerve. Once the olecranon fossa is well visualized, a burr is placed posterolaterally and the

FIGURE 4

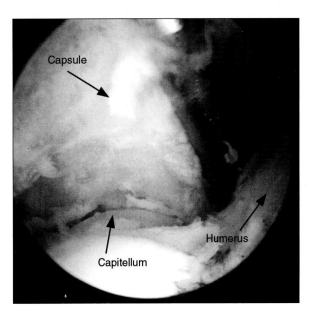

Switching stick in the proximal anterolateral portal used to bluntly sweep the anterior capsule off the distal humerus to create a larger working space.

scope is redirected into the posterior portal. Osteophytes within the fossa are then removed using a round burr. Because the olecranon fossa is oval and not circular, care must be taken to extend the débridement medially and laterally. Often, a posteromedial portal established in a blunt fashion is helpful to place a blunt retractor and maintain the ulnar nerve out of harm's way.

Olecranon tip osteophytes are débrided. This can be an extensive débridement because osteophytes often extend deep into the medial and lateral gutters. Inspection with the arthroscope in the posterocentral portal and the retractor in the posteromedial portal will provide excellent visualization of the medial gutter. Often, the humeral origin of the posterior bundle of the medial collateral ligament can be easily visualized. This can be released sharply off the humerus using a multipolar cautery device set at a low setting and using very short bursts of energy to avoid any thermal injury to the overlying ulnar nerve. Using a retractor, the ulnar nerve is kept superficially away from the area of débridement and a burr is placed down the medial gutter to remove proximal olecranon osteophytes.

Alternatively, if the patient has had a substantial loss of flexion requiring release of the medial collateral ligament and ulnar nerve, a small 2- to 3-cm incision can be made over the ulnar nerve to release the cubital tunnel retinaculum, retract the nerve away from the floor of the cubital tunnel, and then release the posterior bundle of the medial collateral ligament sharply with an open exposure. This can also allow limited access to the most medial of the olecranon osteophytes. This method is recommended early in a surgeon's learning curve. The posterolateral osteophytes are then removed by placing the arthroscope centrally and the burr in the posterolateral portal. With the elbow extended, osteophytes are removed down toward the lateral gutter. After removal of most of the osteophytes using a round burr, the olecranon fossa itself can be further débrided using a rear-entry acorn burr. A 12-mm rear entry acorn burr generally used on anterior cruciate ligament reconstruction is used. This burr can be inserted into the posterior portal with only a small extension of the skin wound. A 12-mm burr often fits quite well into the olecranon fossa, and further débridement toward the coronoid fossa anteriorly using this burr usually accomplishes a very complete bony resection.

Posterolateral Arthroscopy

Finally, posterolateral arthroscopy is performed by placing the scope in the posterolateral portal and the débriding instrument in the midlateral portal. Osteophytes on the posterior capitellum just posterior to the articular surface are débrided in this fashion. Adhesions or plicae are also removed around the radial head. In cases of loss of pronation and supination, removal of adhesions in this location generally results in some improvement.

Wound Closure

The portals are then closed in a figure-of-8 fashion. Multiple sutures are used so that watertight closure is obtained because the subcutaneous location of the elbow joint makes the wound susceptible to drainage. Usually the sutures are not removed for a minimum of 2 weeks, and postoperative oral antibiotics are administered to prevent infection at the portal sites.

POSTOPERATIVE REHABILITATION

The arm is placed in a double-layered compressive dressing with an anterior splint. Usually the arm is wrapped in a single layer of compressive elastic bandage, followed by an anterior splint, and finally a second layer of elastic bandage. The patient is instructed to keep the arm elevated in this extension-immobilized position for a minimum of 24 hours following surgery. After 24 hours, the patient removes the first layer of elastic bandage and the anterior splint, after which a home program of range-of-motion exercises is begun. In our experience, after 24 hours of immobilization and extension with the arm elevated, postoperative swelling is generally minimal. This edema control greatly facilitates range-of-motion exercises following the immobilization.

Active, active-assisted, and passive elbow flexion, extension, supination, and pronation exercises are started after splint removal. Sutures are removed at a 2-week follow-up visit. Nonsteroidal anti-inflammatory drugs are continued from the time of surgery until 6 weeks postoperatively. Maintaining motion is the principal goal of therapy for the initial 6 weeks, and the patient should perform motion exercises every 2 to 3 hours throughout the day. Some authors report that continous passive motion (CPM) is extremely helpful in maintaining early motion after surgery and often continue CPM use throughout the initial postoperative month.[9] Nevertheless, there is no literature supporting the beneficial use of CPM after débridement, and we do not use it. A removable, nighttime anterior extension splint is used to limit loss of extension during the initial postoperative period. Elbow flexor/extensor and forearm supinator/pronator strengthening (isometrics and light resistive exercise) is initiated at 6 weeks and continued for the following 6 weeks.

PEARLS AND PITFALLS

As with any arthroscopic procedure, correct setup and portal placement is critical to being able to efficiently and effectively accomplish the surgical goals, and this is especially true with this demanding arthroscopic procedure. In terms of patient positioning, we recommend the lateral decubitus position because it allows easy access to the posterior compartment without any requirement for specialized holders to stabilize the arm. Critical points when positioning patients in the lateral decubitus position include moving the chest as close to the edge of the table as possible to provide clearance for the elbow to flex fully without abutment and making sure to position the arm at 90° of abduction (perpendicular to the chest). A common mistake is placing the arm in slightly less abduction, which compromises anterior compartment access through the medial portal because instruments or the camera will abut the chest wall. Finally, the opposite arm should be placed on an arm board, positioned abducted slightly higher than the down shoulder. Again, this allows clearance of the hand during full flexion.

For portal placement, we routinely use the anteromedial and anterolateral portals for anterior compartment access. The more proximal the anterolateral portal, the more difficult it is to gain access to the medial portion of the anterior compartment for débridement of the coronoid tip or the coronoid fossa. This problem is exacerbated in the setting of arthritis with prominent osteophytes along the anterolateral distal humeral supracondylar ridge. Consequently, we recommend placing the anterolateral portal slightly more distal to gain medial access. As long as the portal is not placed distal to the radiocapitellar joint, it can be considered safe with regard to the radial nerve.

Retractors can significantly aid in visualization and safety during the procedure. Anteriorly, two lateral portals may be established, allowing a retractor in one and the camera or a working instrument in the other. Posteriorly, a second posterocentral portal placed a few centimeters proximal to the first can also be used for retractor placement, keeping the posterior joint capsule medially (along with the ulnar nerve) away from burrs or shavers.

Arthroscopic osteocapsular arthroplasty is a complex and difficult operation, and surgeons should recognize their limitations and be willing to convert to an open procedure if necessary. Results of open débridement are predictable; therefore, the surgeon should not compromise safety. It is recommended that the surgeon gain experience with this procedure by "working up to it" by performing several simpler operations to gain arthroscopic experience. Simpler procedures include diagnostic arthroscopies, loose body removals, and lateral epicondylitis releases.

Proper instrumentation can improve the efficiency and effectiveness of the procedure. A small-joint arthroscope is not required for this procedure, but we recommend having an assortment of different sizes and shapes of shavers and burrs available. The burr sizes should be approximately 4 mm and they all should be hooded. An assortment of round, cone-shaped, and tapered heads makes it easier to remove bone. Curved shavers can also be used to gain access from a lateral portal to the medial aspect of the joint. A cautery/tissue ablator device is extremely helpful to clear soft tissue efficiently. The surgeon should understand that excess heat in a small space can pose a risk to cartilage and surrounding nerves; therefore, we advise setting the heat level at half of what is routinely used for a larger joint to limit the effects of excessive heat.

OUTCOMES OF TREATMENT

Open and arthroscopic treatment of elbow arthritis have both shown predictable improvements in pain relief, motion, and functional outcomes at mid- to long-term follow-up. Proposed advantages of arthroscopic treatment include less surgical morbidity and shorter recovery times. Limitations of arthroscopic débridement include the inability to perform as complete of a release or débridement because of technical challenges and concern for neurologic injury. Despite these potential limitations, early results of arthroscopic treatment do not suggest that it is associated with an increased risk of complications or that it fails to achieve improvements in motion, pain, and function.

Morrey[3] reported on 15 patients at a mean follow-up of 33 months after open ulnohumeral arthroplasty. The elbow flexion extension arc improved a mean of 21°, and 80% of patients had a good or excellent result as defined by the Mayo Elbow Performance Score (MEPS). Antuna and associates[10] reported longer term outcomes in 46 patients treated at the Mayo Clinic with ulnohumeral arthroplasty for primary degenerative elbow arthritis. At a mean of 80 months postoperatively, 76% of patients had a good or excellent result on the MEPS with an average improvement in flexion arc of 22°; however, 29% of patients reported postoperative ulnar nerve symptoms. Phillips and associates[11] evaluated 20 patients with the Disabilities of the Arm, Shoulder and Hand (DASH) questionnaire and the MEPS at a mean of 75 months postoperatively and reported 65% good or excellent results by the MEPS and only 40% of patients with DASH scores <20. Tashjian and associates[12] reported more optimistic functional outcome scores after open ulnohumeral arthroplasty at an average of 85 months, with 83% good or excellent results by the MEPS, 94% of patients having DASH scores <20, and average Short Form-36 (SF-36) scores better than age- and sex-adjusted normal values. Overall, open ulnohumeral arthroplasty provides durable improvements in pain, motion (~20° flexion arc), and physician-derived (MEPS) and patient-derived (DASH, SF-36) functional outcomes at long term.

Outcomes of arthroscopic treatment of elbow arthritis also have been reported. Redden and Stanley[6] initially reported satisfactory results of arthroscopic fenestration alone, with improvements in pain but no improvements in motion. Cohen and associates[13] performed open Outerbridge-Kashiwagi procedures and arthroscopic fenestrations (as described by Redden and Stanley[6]) in 44 patients (18 Outerbridge-Kashiwagi procedures and 26 arthroscopic fenestrations). In this series, arthroscopic débridement and fenestration provided better pain relief than open Outerbridge-Kashiwagi procedures, while Outerbridge-Kashiwagi procedures provided significantly greater improvements in flexion-extension arc. Ogilvie-Harris and associates[5] reported on 25 patients a mean of 35 months after arthroscopic posterior débridement (osteophytes, loose bodies, olecranon tip) with humeral fenestration. Pain, function, and motion significantly improved from baseline, with more than 50% of patients obtaining full extension at follow-up. Savoie and associates[7] were the first to report on a "complete" arthroscopic débridement, including anterior and posterior compartments with complete capsular release and humeral fenestration. Twenty-four patients were evaluated an average of 32 months postoperatively and were found to have significant improvements in pain along with an average of 81° improvement in flexion arc. Recently, Krishnan and associates[14] reported similar results in patients younger than 50 years of age who were treated with the same surgical procedure as Savoie and associates, with significant improvements in pain and satisfaction. The average flexion arc improved an average of 71°. Kelly and associates[15] also reported on complete arthroscopic débridement in 25 elbows in which sharp capsular release was not performed. At an average of 67 months, 84% of patients were found to have a good or excellent result, although the flexion arc improved by an average of only 21°. No neurologic complications were reported in any arthroscopic series.[7,14,15] Although 75% of the patients in the Savoie series underwent radial head resection, almost no patients in the series of Krishnan and associates[14] and Kelly and associates[15] underwent concomitant resection, calling into question the necessity of this component of the procedure.

Both open and arthroscopic elbow débridement provide mid-term improvements in pain and functional improvements in patients with moderate degenerative arthritis. The addition of a sharp capsular release, which is not part of the reported results of the open ulnohumeral arthroplasty, appears to significantly improve the flexion arc. The two studies including a sharp anterior and posterior capsular release, Krishnan and associates[14] and Savoie and associates,[7] report approximately 50° to 60° greater improvement in flexion arc than either open or arthroscopic procedures not including a sharp capsular release. It is unclear whether transhumeral fenestration is required to produce and maintain improvements in pain and motion if re-creation of normal anatomy with bony débridement and complete capsular release alone is performed. It is also unclear whether radial head resection is required, even when grade III or IV radiocapitellar arthritis is present. Finally, there appears to be no increased risk of surgical complications, including neurovascular injury, with arthroscopic compared to open procedures in experienced hands. Further research is required to determine the long-term

(>10-year) durability of arthroscopic osteocapsular arthroplasty with regard to functional outcome and radiographic progression of arthritis. Keeping these limitations in mind, arthroscopic osteocapsular arthroplasty is a reliable surgical treatment of both young and older patients with moderate degenerative elbow arthritis.

REFERENCES

1. Morrey BF: Primary degenerative arthritis of the elbow: Ulnohumeral arthroplasty, in Morrey BF (ed): *The Elbow and Its Disorders*, ed 3. Philadelphia, PA, Saunders, 2000, pp 74-83.

2. Kashiwagi D: Intra-articular changes of the osteoarthritic elbow, especially about the fossa olecrani. *Jpn Orthop Assoc* 1978;52:1367-1372.

3. Morrey BF: Primary degenerative arthritis of the elbow: Treatment by ulnohumeral arthroplasty. *J Bone Joint Surg Br* 1992;74:409-413.

4. O'Driscoll SW: Arthroscopic treatment for osteoarthritis of the elbow. *Orthop Clin North Am* 1995;26:691-706.

5. Ogilvie-Harris DJ, Gordon R, MacKay M: Arthroscopic treatment for posterior impingement in degenerative arthritis of the elbow. *Arthroscopy* 1995;11:437-443.

6. Redden JF, Stanley D: Arthroscopic fenestration of the olecranon fossa in the treatment of osteoarthritis of the elbow. *Arthroscopy* 1993;9:14-16.

7. Savoie FH, Nunley PD, Field LD: Arthroscopic management of the arthritic elbow: Indications, technique, and results. *J Shoulder Elbow Surg* 1999;8:214-219.

8. Yamaguchi K, Tashjian RZ: Setup and portals, in Yamaguchi K, King GJW, McKee MD, O'Driscoll SW (eds): *Advanced Reconstruction Elbow*. Rosemont, IL, American Academy of Orthopaedic Surgeons, 2007, pp 3-11.

9. O'Driscoll SW: Arthroscopic osteocapsular arthroplasty, in Yamaguchi K, King GJW, McKee MD, O'Driscoll SW (eds): *Advanced Reconstruction Elbow*. Rosemont, IL, American Academy of Orthopaedic Surgeons, 2007, pp 59-68.

10. Antuna SA, Morrey BF, Adams RA, O'Driscoll SW: Ulnohumeral arthroplasty for primary degenerative arthritis of the elbow: Long-term outcome and complications. *J Bone Joint Surg Am* 2002;84:2168-2173.

11. Phillips NJ, Ali A, Stanley D: Treatment of primary degenerative arthritis of the elbow by ulnohumeral arthroplasty: A long-term follow-up. *J Bone Joint Surg Br* 2003;85:347-350.

12. Tashjian RZ, Wolf JM, Ritter M, Weiss AP, Green A: Functional outcomes and general health status after ulnohumeral arthroplasty for primary degenerative arthritis of the elbow. *J Shoulder Elbow Surg* 2006;15:357-366.

13. Cohen AP, Redden JF, Stanley D: Treatment of osteoarthritis of the elbow: A comparison of open and arthroscopic debridement. *Arthroscopy* 2000;16:701-706.

14. Krishnan SG, Harkins DC, Pennington SD, Harrison DK, Burkhead WZ: Arthroscopic ulnohumeral arthroplasty for degenerative arthritis of the elbow in patients under fifty years of age. *J Shoulder Elbow Surg* 2007;16:443-448.

15. Kelly EW, Bryce R, Coghlan J, Bell S: Arthroscopic debridement without radial head excision of the osteoarthritic elbow. *Arthroscopy* 2007;23:151-156.

INDEX

Page numbers followed by *f* indicate figures; page numbers followed by *t* indicate tables.